MUSCULOSKELETAL FUNCTION

Musculoskeletal Function: An Anatomy and Kinesiology Laboratory Manual

by Dortha Esch and Marvin Lepley

Illustrations by Jean Magney

UNIVERSITY OF MINNESOTA PRESS

MINNEAPOLIS

Printed in the United States of America at
the University of Minnesota Printing Department.

Published in the United Kingdom and India by the Oxford
University Press, London and Delhi.

Library of Congress Catalog Card Number: 73-93577
ISBN 0-8166-0716-8

Second printing, 1976

Preface

This manual was prepared as a guide for study of the way the musculo-skeletal system functions and of kinesiology, which are vital subjects for the therapist, physical educator, and others interested in motor function. The motivation to write it came from our desire to increase the relevance of this important subject matter by combining the structural detail of anatomy with the interesting study of function. An additional benefit we discovered is that it enables students to work more independently in the classroom, thus resulting in an economic use of faculty time. When the manual is used one instructor can effectively supervise thirty or more students. The interest of the student is maintained by the variety of study methods incorporated: surface anatomy, the analysis of muscle actions, the analysis of activities, and the problems which bring in the mechanical aspects of motor function.

The manual includes sections on osteology, skeletal landmarks, surface anatomy, and kinesiology, the latter providing a guide for the study of muscle actions. The section on surface anatomy gives directions for location and palpation of muscles on a subject. This approach to study is seldom found in an anatomy or kinesiology text. The final section is devoted to problems which help the student learn the effect of mechanics on motor function as well as the ways in which muscles work together to provide coordinated movement. Some of the problems are directed to the analysis of simple activities.

The illustrations were designed to depict function rather than anatomic structure as found in anatomy texts. That is, the view and position of the skeletal part were selected to demonstrate function. The muscle illustrations were cut from Zip-A-Tone screen in order to show graphically the layers of muscles on one drawing.

Previous versions of the manual have been used in the classroom for four years, with improvements made each year and new sections added. Although it would be possible to use the manual as an exclusive text, it was not so intended. In addition to it, we use Functional Anatomy of the Limbs and Back by W. Henry Hollinshead and Clinical Kinesiology by Signe Brunnstrom.

Beyond its use in the classroom the manual may serve the professional needing a quick review of anatomy and kinesiology.

At the University of Minnesota the manual is used as a guide for the students in the kinesiology laboratory which is a part of the functional anatomy course. This course was developed during a curriculum revision three years ago in response to a concern we felt regarding the increasing volume of subject matter required in the education of an occupational therapist. We combined two courses which were five credits each into one six-credit course. The new course comprises lecture and demonstration, an anatomy laboratory (with prosected human cadavers), and a kinesiology laboratory, which includes the study of surface anatomy and the analysis of actions and activities. After two years' experience with the new course we found no decrease in learning among students and, in fact, an increase in the enthusiasm of students for working with the material.

We would like to thank our colleagues who provided help and offered encouragement during the development of this manual. A number of individuals have given invaluable assistance including our occupational therapy students, who while using the early drafts of the manual provided feedback in many ways, and the occupational therapy faculty at the University of Minnesota who consulted with us and gave us moral support when it was needed. We are indebted to John D. Allison, R.P.T., Martin O. Mundale, R.P.T., and James F. Pohtilla, R.P.T., who have shared their knowledge of the subject matter.

Special recognition and thanks go to those who have read parts of the manuscript and have given us the benefit of their constructive criticism: Shelby Clayson, R.P.T., and A. Joy Huss, O.T.R., R.P.T. Last, but no means least, we thank Darlene Kriska and Barbara Bartholomew, who spent many hours typing and proofreading the manuscript and who provided helpful suggestions for the format.

The preparation of the manual was assisted financially, in part, by S.R.S. Grant No. 16-P-56810, awarded to the Regional Rehabilitation Research and Training Center, RT-2, at the University of Minnesota Medical School.

Dortha Esch, B.S., O.T.R.
Marvin Lepley, B.S., O.T.R.

University of Minnesota
October 1973

Contents

MUSCULOSKELETAL FUNCTION

Osteology

Introduction

The study of osteology is a necessary first step in the development of an understanding of human motion. The skeletal system provides the structure of the musculoskeletal system, with the bones joined in a variety of articulations which allow different kinds of movement. Since the skeleton provides the points of attachment for the muscles, which provide the force for motion, knowledge of the bony landmarks is essential for determining their line of action. The landmarks designated on the following pages are those which are most important for the analysis of motion.

Suggested procedure for study:

1. Look at each bone. Note its position in relation to the body.

2. Study the articular surfaces of each bone. The shape of the articular surfaces is one factor which determines the type of motions that will be possible as well as the amount of motion in any given plane.

3. Identify each designated landmark and note its relationship to nearby joints. The relationship of landmarks to joints determines the effective motion produced by a muscle as it applies force to the landmark.

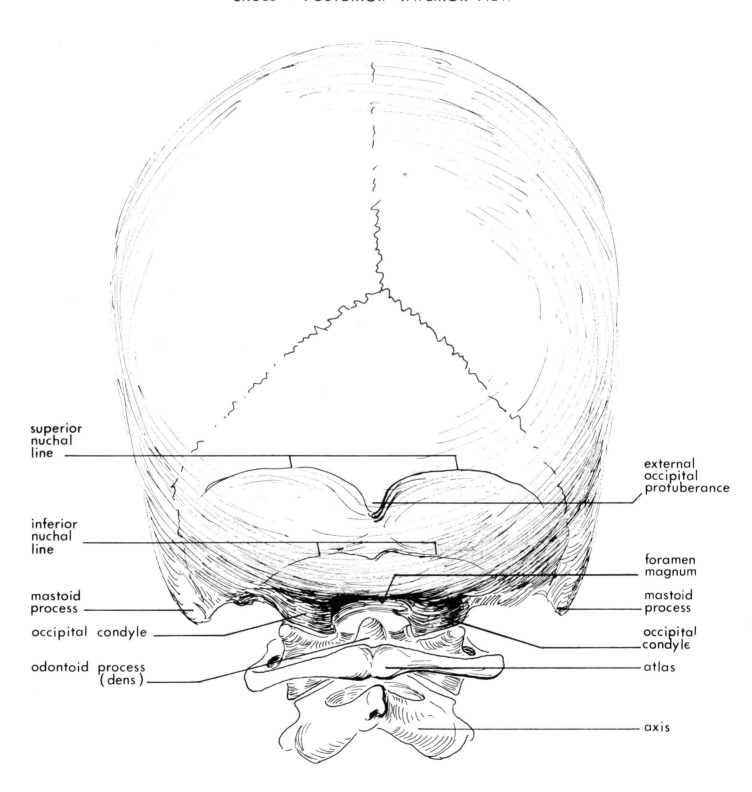

superior
nuchal
line

external
occipital
protuberance

inferior
nuchal
line

mastoid
process

foramen
magnum

mastoid
process

occipital condyle

occipital
condyle

odontoid process
(dens)

atlas

axis

4

TYPICAL VERTEBRAE

Cervical

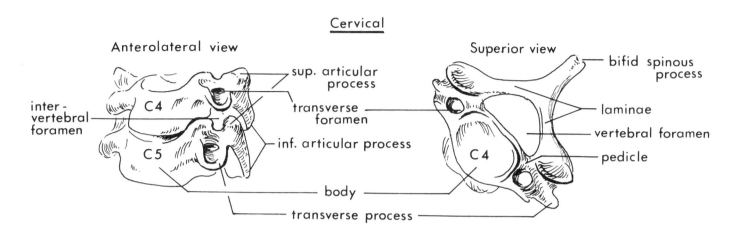

Anterolateral view

Superior view

inter-vertebral foramen

sup. articular process

transverse foramen

inf. articular process

body

transverse process

C4

C5

bifid spinous process

laminae

vertebral foramen

pedicle

C4

Thoracic

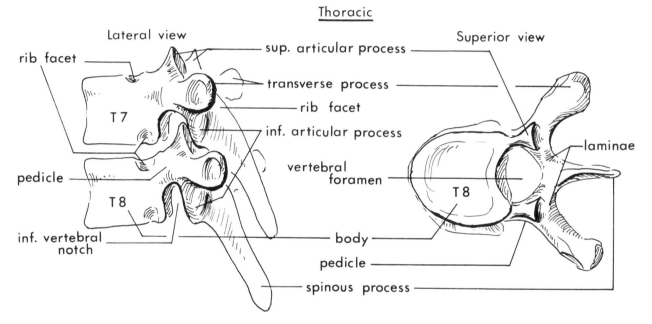

Lateral view

Superior view

rib facet

pedicle

inf. vertebral notch

sup. articular process

transverse process

rib facet

inf. articular process

vertebral foramen

body

pedicle

spinous process

T7

T8

T8

laminae

Lumbar

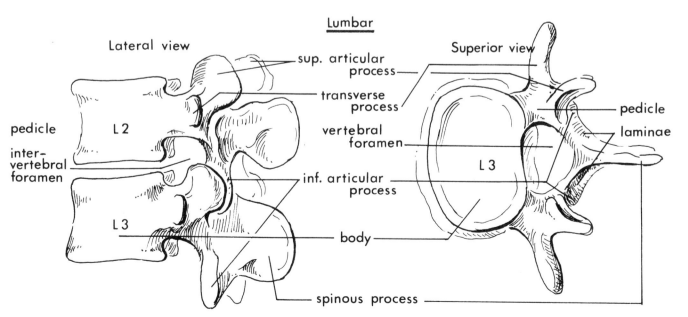

Lateral view

Superior view

pedicle

inter-vertebral foramen

sup. articular process

transverse process

vertebral foramen

inf. articular process

body

spinous process

L2

L3

L3

pedicle

laminae

ATLANTOAXIAL ARTICULATION

odontoid process ———————

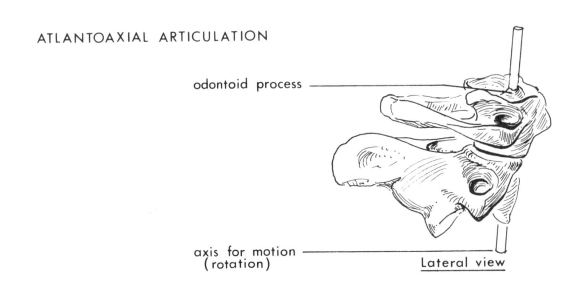

axis for motion
(rotation) ———————

Lateral view

odontoid process

articular facet (occipital)

axis for motion
(flexion - extension)

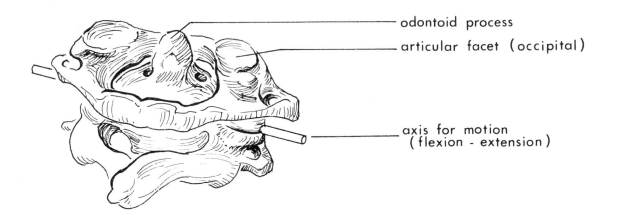

Posterolateral view

articular facet (occipital) ———————
odontoid process ———————

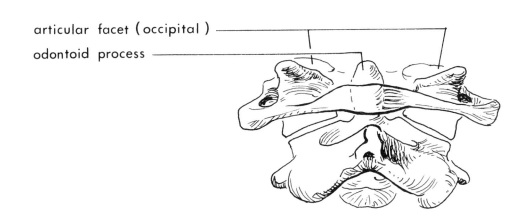

Posterior view

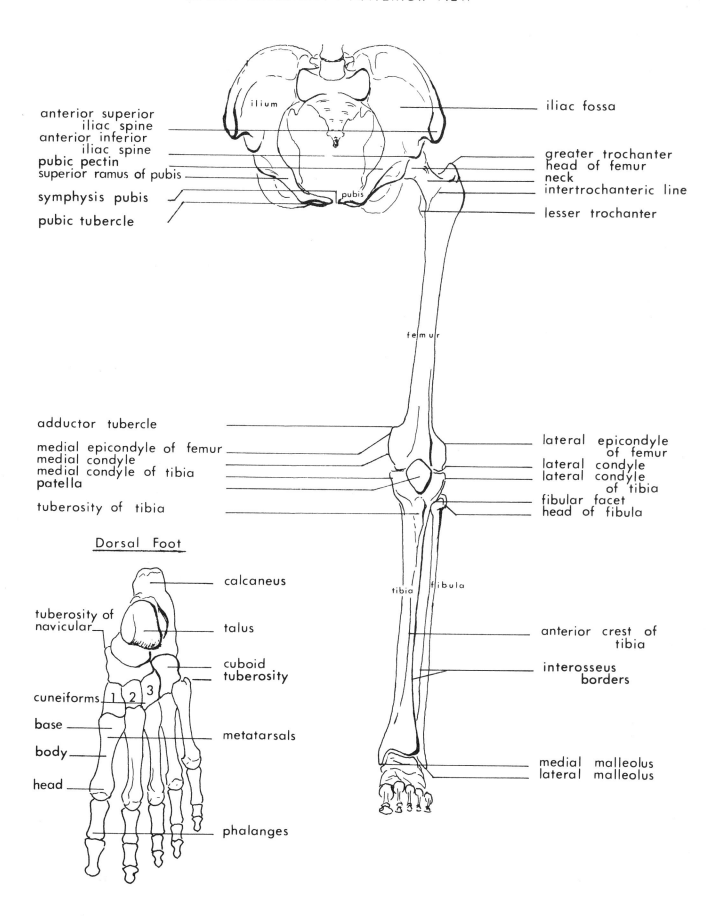

anterior superior
iliac spine

anterior inferior
iliac spine

pubic pectin

superior ramus of pubis

symphysis pubis

pubic tubercle

ilium

pubis

iliac fossa

greater trochanter
head of femur
neck
intertrochanteric line

lesser trochanter

femur

adductor tubercle

medial epicondyle of femur
medial condyle
medial condyle of tibia
patella

tuberosity of tibia

lateral epicondyle
of femur
lateral condyle
lateral condyle
of tibia
fibular facet
head of fibula

Dorsal Foot

calcaneus

tuberosity of
navicular

talus

cuboid
tuberosity

cuneiforms 1 2 3

base

body

head

metatarsals

phalanges

tibia   fibula

anterior crest of
tibia

interosseus
borders

medial malleolus
lateral malleolus

7

LOWER EXTREMITY : POSTERIOR VIEW

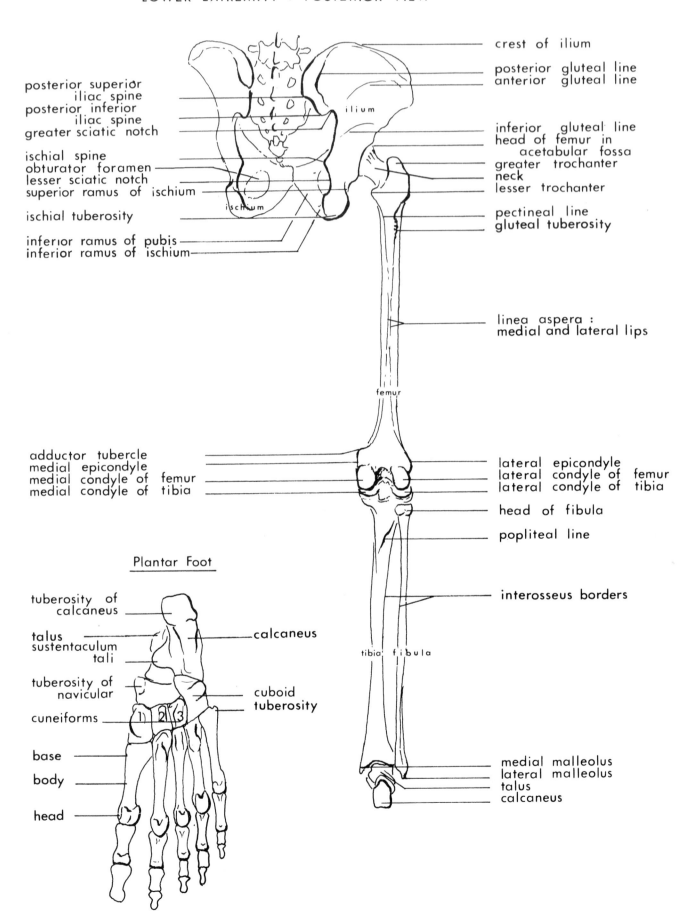

crest of ilium

posterior gluteal line
anterior gluteal line

ilium

posterior superior
iliac spine
posterior inferior
iliac spine
greater sciatic notch

inferior gluteal line
head of femur in
acetabular fossa
greater trochanter
neck
lesser trochanter

ischial spine
obturator foramen
lesser sciatic notch
superior ramus of ischium

ischium

pectineal line
gluteal tuberosity

ischial tuberosity

inferior ramus of pubis
inferior ramus of ischium

linea aspera :
medial and lateral lips

femur

adductor tubercle
medial epicondyle
medial condyle of femur
medial condyle of tibia

lateral epicondyle
lateral condyle of femur
lateral condyle of tibia

head of fibula

popliteal line

Plantar Foot

tuberosity of
calcaneus

interosseus borders

talus
sustentaculum
tali

calcaneus

tuberosity of
navicular

cuboid
tuberosity

cuneiforms

1 2 3

tibia fibula

base

body

medial malleolus
lateral malleolus
talus
calcaneus

head

UPPER EXTREMITY : POSTERIOR VIEW

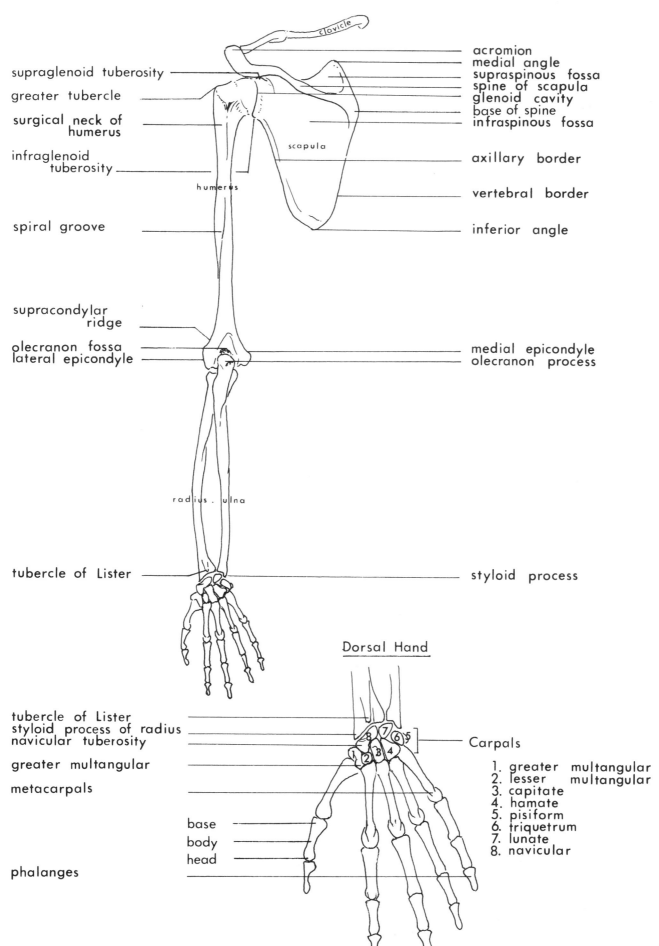

clavicle

acromion
medial angle
supraspinous fossa
spine of scapula
glenoid cavity
base of spine
infraspinous fossa

supraglenoid tuberosity

greater tubercle

surgical neck of
humerus

infraglenoid
tuberosity

axillary border

scapula

vertebral border

humerus

spiral groove

inferior angle

supracondylar
ridge

olecranon fossa
lateral epicondyle

medial epicondyle
olecranon process

radius . ulna

tubercle of Lister

styloid process

Dorsal Hand

tubercle of Lister
styloid process of radius
navicular tuberosity

Carpals

greater multangular

metacarpals

1. greater multangular
2. lesser multangular
3. capitate
4. hamate
5. pisiform
6. triquetrum
7. lunate
8. navicular

base
body
head

phalanges

9

UPPER EXTREMITY : ANTERIOR VIEW

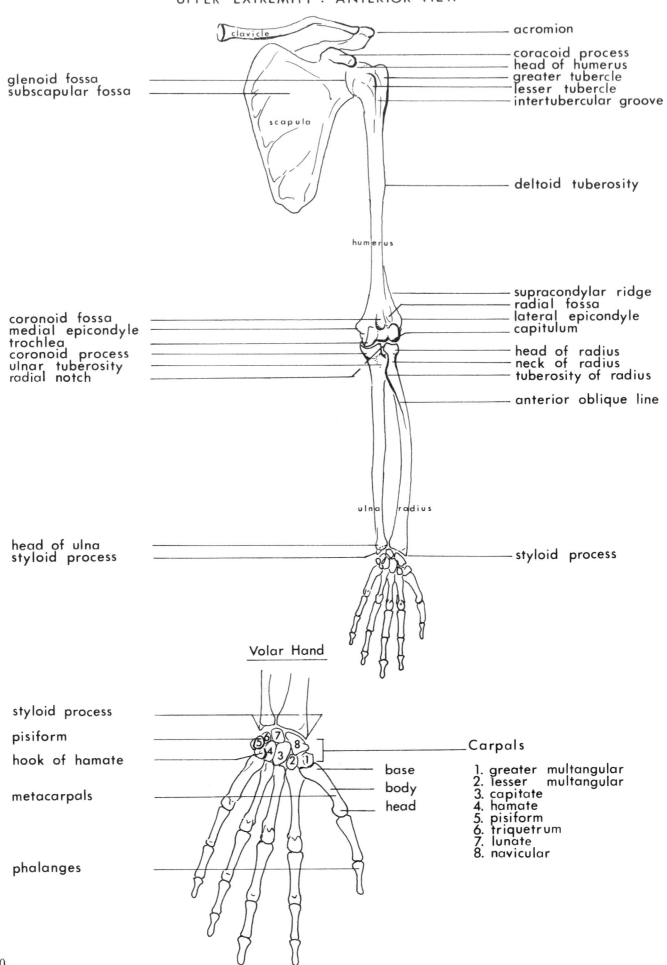

clavicle

acromion
coracoid process
head of humerus
greater tubercle
lesser tubercle
intertubercular groove

glenoid fossa
subscapular fossa

scapula

deltoid tuberosity

humerus

supracondylar ridge
radial fossa
lateral epicondyle
capitulum

coronoid fossa
medial epicondyle
trochlea
coronoid process
ulnar tuberosity
radial notch

head of radius
neck of radius
tuberosity of radius

anterior oblique line

ulna   radius

head of ulna
styloid process

styloid process

Volar Hand

styloid process

pisiform

hook of hamate

metacarpals

phalanges

base
body
head

Carpals

1. greater multangular
2. lesser multangular
3. capitate
4. hamate
5. pisiform
6. triquetrum
7. lunate
8. navicular

10

Skeletal Landmarks

Introduction

The skeletal landmarks included in this section are those which are relatively easy to identify on yourself or a subject. The ability to locate these landmarks is a necessary first step for the identification of muscles. It will also help you relate your knowledge of anatomy to your own body and will facilitate your understanding of the function of the musculoskeletal system.

Recommended procedure for study of this section:

1. Identify the bony landmarks on the skeleton. The osteology charts in this manual may be used as a reference.

2. Read the directions for locating the skeletal landmark and palpate or observe it on your subject.

Your study and analysis of motion will be facilitated if you develop an awareness of the relationship of the landmarks to each other and to the joint or joints in that anatomic area.

Pelvis, Thigh, and Knee

ILIUM

CREST: The crest may be easily palpated or seen on most subjects. The highest point on the crest is at the level of the spinous process of the fourth lumbar vertebra.

ANTERIOR SUPERIOR ILIAC SPINE (ASIS): Trace the crest forward to its most anterior point, which is the rounded ASIS.

POSTERIOR SUPERIOR ILIAC SPINE (PSIS): Follow the crest posteriorly to this prominence, which is about one and one-half inches from the midline of the back. On many subjects a small depression will be seen at the site of the PSIS.

SACRUM: Palpate the flat bone at the center of the back between the posterior spines of the two ilia.

ISCHIUM

TUBEROSITY: This large bony prominence is most easily palpated at the midline of the buttock with your subject in a sitting position. This is often called the "sit bone" and, for patients who lack sensation, is a potential area for the development of decubitus ulcers.

PUBIS

SYMPHYSIS: This is the area where the two pubic bones join.

FEMUR

GREATER TROCHANTER: This is a large prominence which may be palpated about four to five inches inferior to the most lateral portion of the iliac crest. It will be found in the depression that appears when the thigh is abducted. You will feel the prominence move during internal and external rotation of the thigh.

MEDIAL AND LATERAL CONDYLES: With the knee flexed these are easily palpated on either side of the patella (kneecap).

ADDUCTOR TUBERCLE: This prominence may be difficult to identify on some subjects. Palpate with deep pressure on the superior medial margin of the medial condyle.

PATELLA: This is a sesamoid bone which is easily seen and palpated. If the knee is in the extended position with the leg supported, it becomes freely movable because the quadriceps muscle is relaxed. The patella increases the leverage of the knee extensor muscles.

TIBIA

MEDIAL AND LATERAL CONDYLES: With the knee flexed, palpate just inferior to the femoral condyles.

TUBEROSITY: With the knee flexed, the prominence may be easily palpated approximately two inches below the inferior border of the patella.

FIBULA

HEAD: Palpate at the posterolateral aspect of the lateral condyle of the tibia, at the level of the tibial tuberosity.

Leg and Foot

ANTERIOR BORDER (CREST) OF THE TIBIA: Observe or palpate from tibial tuberosity to the ankle.

MALLEOLI: Palpate at the distal end of the tibia and fibula. Note that the lateral malleolus is more inferior and posterior.

CALCANEUS: Palpate on the medial and lateral sides of the heel.

TUBEROSITY OF THE FIFTH METATARSAL: Palpate at the base, proximal end, of the fifth metatarsal. It forms the most lateral projection on the foot.

CUBOID: Palpate in the depression just posterior to the tuberosity of the fifth metatarsal.

SUSTENTACULUM TALUS: Palpate about an inch below the medial malleolus. This projection of the calcaneus forms a shelf on which part of the talus rests.

FIRST METATARSAL: Palpate on the medial or dorsal surface of the foot.

TUBEROSITY OF THE NAVICULAR: Palpate on the medial surface of the navicular, just posterior to the first metatarsal.

Shoulder Girdle and Arm

CLAVICLE

STERNAL END: Palpate the rounded projection above the superior aspect of the manubrium sterni. The depression found between the sternal ends of the two clavicles is called the suprasternal notch or fossa.

SHAFT: Palpate the anterior and superior surfaces from medial to lateral. Note that the anterior surface is convex medially and concave laterally.

ACROMIAL END: This prominence of the lateral end of the clavicle, which articulates with the acromion process of the scapula and projects above it, is easily palpable.

SCAPULA

INFERIOR ANGLE: Palpate the lowest portion of the scapula, which is the junction of the medial and lateral borders. If your subject consciously relaxes the shoulder girdle musculature, the angle will be more easily palpated.

MEDIAL (VERTEBRAL) BORDER: This border is easily palpated about one and one-half inches lateral to the vertebrae.

LATERAL (AXILLARY) BORDER: With the arm and shoulder relaxed, the border may be palpated from the inferior angle to the axilla.

ACROMION PROCESS: Palpate this flat process at the lateral point of the shoulder where it forms a shelf over the glenohumeral joint.

SPINE: Palpate from the acromion process to its base on the vertebral border.

CORACOID PROCESS: Palpate with deep pressure through the medial border of the anterior deltoid muscle, just inferior to the clavicular concavity. If you have difficulty, ask your subject to protract his shoulder slightly.

Note: Study the general shape and placement of the scapula with the body in anatomic position. Note that on the skeleton it is located between the second and the seventh ribs.

HUMERUS

GREATER TUBERCLE: With the arm in internal rotation, palpate just distal to the anterior portion of the acromion process. As your subject internally rotates his arm you will feel it move under your fingers.

LESSER TUBERCLE: With the humerus in external rotation, palpate anterior to the greater tubercle.

INTERTUBERCULAR GROOVE: Palpate between the greater and the lesser tubercles.

EPICONDYLES, MEDIAL AND LATERAL: With the forearm extended, palpate in the upper part of medial and lateral fossae on the posterior surface of the elbow. Also, locate the ulnar nerve in the medial fossa between the olecranon process and the medial epicondyle.

Forearm, Wrist, and Hand

The bony prominences are numbered on the drawings and the same number, in parentheses, appears in the text following the name of the prominence.

ULNA

OLECRANON PROCESS: This large process, the proximal end of the ulna, is easily palpated on the dorsal surface of the elbow joint.

BODY: On the dorsal surface of the forearm, palpate the body (shaft) of the ulna from the olecranon process to the distal end or head.

HEAD (1): The head may be seen as a rounded projection on the dorsal surface of the forearm.

STYLOID PROCESS (2): Palpate this small projection on the medial aspect of the head of the ulna. With your subject's forearm in pronation, place one finger on the styloid and ask him to supinate. Note the changing position of the styloid as the ulna rotates.

RADIUS

HEAD: With the elbow extended, palpate on the dorsal surface just distal to the lateral condyle of the humerus. With one finger on the radial head, ask your subject to pronate and supinate the forearm; note its rotation.

STYLOID PROCESS (3): Palpate on the lateral aspect of the wrist, proximal to the first metacarpal.

TUBERCLE OF LISTER (4): Palpate on the dorsum of the radius about one inch laterally from the head of the ulna. The tendon of the extensor pollicis longus lies on the ulnar side of this prominence.

Locate the radial tuberosity on the skeleton and note its rotation as the forearm is pronated and supinated.

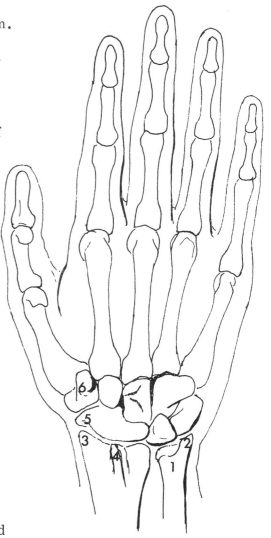

DORSAL SURFACE

CARPALS

NAVICULAR TUBEROSITY (5): Palpate just distal to the styloid process of the radius, on the floor of the anatomic snuffbox (the triangular shaped depression between the extensor pollicis longus and brevis tendons).

GREATER MULTANGULAR (6): Palpate on the floor of the anatomic snuffbox, proximal to the first metacarpal.

PISIFORM (7): Palpate on the palmar side of the wrist on the ulnar border, just distal to the distal wrist crease. Abduction of the little finger against resistance will cause contraction of the flexor carpi ulnaris muscle, and this will make the pisiform more prominent.

HOOK OF THE HAMATE (8): With deep pressure, palpate on the medial side of the hand, at about the middle of the hypothenar eminence.

METACARPALS: Palpate the body, head, and base on the dorsum of the hand.

PHALANGES: Palpate on the dorsum of the fingers.

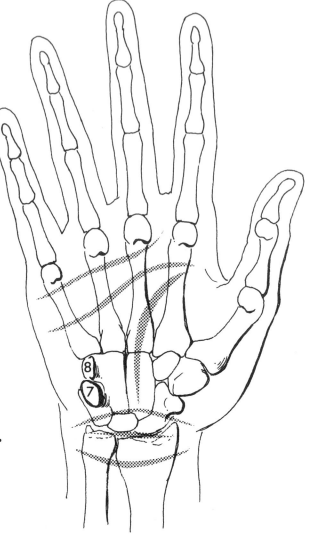

PALMAR SURFACE

WRIST CREASES: With the wrist in about 45 degrees of flexion note the three creases. The most distal is at the proximal edge of the flexor retinaculum (transverse carpal ligament), the middle is at the level of the articulation between the proximal row of carpals and the radius, and the proximal is at the proximal end of the synovial sheaths of the flexor tendons.

PALMAR CREASES: Identify the midpalmar and thenar creases.

16

Surface Anatomy

Introduction

The muscles included in this section are those which can be observed or palpated with relative ease. Many deep muscles are difficult or impossible to identify on a subject with normal musculature. The ability to identify the muscles on yourself or a classmate will increase your understanding of their actions. The occupational or physical therapist uses this skill in the evaluation of the patient's motor function.

Recommended procedure for study of this section:

1. Read the directions for identification of the muscle and/or its attachments. Some muscles may be easily seen as they contract, while others are partially covered and only identified through palpation in a specific area.

2. Position your subject as directed.

3. Determine the general area of the muscle by identifying the landmarks listed. The illustrations in the kinesiology section of this manual and those in anatomy or kinesiology textbooks will provide useful references.

4. Ask your subject to perform the motion or motions listed.

5. Apply only moderate resistance as directed. The use of maximum resistance often results in the contraction of many muscles, some of which may obscure the muscle you are trying to identify. In some instances the muscle will be visible or palpable without the use of any resistance.

6. Through palpation or observation identify the muscle. For the comfort of your subject use the tips of several fingers with a medium amount of pressure for palpation. Very light palpation may tickle and very deep pressure, especially over bony prominences, may be painful.

7. As you identify each muscle try to visualize the direction of its fibers and its line of pull in relation to the joint or joints which it crosses.

Neck and Trunk

STERNOCLEIDOMASTOID

Position of Subject: Supine.
Skeletal Landmarks: Superior border of sternum, medial part of clavicle, and mastoid process.
Motions: For one muscle — neck flexion with rotation (for left sterno-cleidomastoid, flex and rotate to the right). For both muscles — neck flexion.
Resistance: Apply resistance to forehead pushing toward extension. For one muscle, apply resistance to the side of the forehead opposite the contracting muscle, pushing in a slightly diagonal direction.

The muscle may be easily seen on the anterolateral surface of the neck.

RECTUS ABDOMINIS

Position of Subject: Supine.
Skeletal Landmarks: Inferior border of sternum and pubis.
Motions: Trunk flexion. Ask your subject to raise his head and shoulders off the table. It is preferable to have your subject flex only enough to clear the scapula from the table. Flexion past this point is primarily performed by the hip flexor muscles.
Resistance: None usually necessary.

The muscles may be palpated as two three-inch-wide bands on either side of the midline of the trunk. On some subjects the three transverse connective tissue bands, called tendinous inscriptions, may be seen.

EXTERNAL AND INTERNAL OBLIQUE ABDOMINIS

Position of Subject: Supine with arms at sides.
Skeletal Landmarks: Anterior crest of ilium, pubis, and anterior aspect of ribs.
Motion: Trunk flexion with rotation. For the right external oblique and the left internal oblique, ask your subject to raise his head and shoulders off the table and point his right shoulder toward his left knee.
Resistance: None usually necessary.

The muscles may be palpated on the anterior and lateral surfaces of the abdomen between the rib cage and the ilium. During trunk rotation the two contracting muscles, the external oblique on one side and the internal oblique on the other, feel like one continuous muscle running in a diagonal direction across the abdomen.

NECK EXTENSOR MUSCLES

Position of Subject: Prone.
Skeletal Landmarks: Cervical vertebrae and occiput.
Motion: Neck extension.
Resistance: Apply resistance on back of skull, pushing toward flexion. The splenius, upper trapezius, and erector spinae muscles may be palpated as a group on either side of the cervical spine.

TRUNK EXTENSOR MUSCLES

Position of Subject: Prone.
Skeletal Landmarks: Thoracic and lumbar vertebrae.
Motion: Back extension. Ask your subject to raise his head and chest off the table.
Resistance: Apply resistance to upper thoracic area, pushing toward flexion.

The muscles may be palpated as a group on either side of the vertebral spines. It should be remembered that these muscles are covered by the superficial muscles of the back which makes detailed identification difficult. The muscle group in the lumbar area is most easily palpated.

Anterior Thigh

SARTORIUS

Position of Subject: Supine.
Skeletal Landmark: Anterior superior iliac spine.
Motion: Hip abduction, flexion, and external rotation. Knee flexion. (Ask your subject to place the heel of the leg being examined on the opposite knee.)
Resistance: Apply resistance above knee, pushing thigh toward extension and adduction.

The sartorius may be easily palpated at the center of the anterior thigh near its attachment to the anterior superior iliac spine. On a few subjects it may be seen as it courses diagonally across the anterior thigh.

TENSOR FASCIA LATAE

Position of Subject: Lying on side.
Skeletal Landmark: Anterior crest of ilium.
Motions: Hip abduction and internal rotation with slight flexion.
Resistance: Apply resistance above knee, pushing thigh toward
   adduction.

Palpate the tensor fascia latae just posterior to the sartorius where it
attaches to the crest of the ilium. Trace the muscle belly to its attachment on the iliotibial band at the junction of the upper and middle thirds
of the thigh. The iliotibial band may be seen or palpated as a hard flat
area on the lateral side of the thigh and is most easily identified just
superior to the knee. If you have difficulty locating the iliotibial band
ask your subject to assume the long sitting position (sitting on the table
with legs extended) and to lift his heel off the table while you palpate on
the lateral inferior aspect of the thigh.

QUADRICEPS FEMORIS

Position of Subject: Supine with leg hanging over end of table.
Skeletal Landmarks: Anterior inferior iliac spine, patella, and tibial
   tuberosity.
Motion: Extension of knee.
Resistance: Apply resistance above ankle, pushing leg toward
   extension.

The three superficial muscles of the quadriceps femoris, the rectus
femoris, vastus lateralis, and vastus medialis, are responsible for the
contour of the anterior thigh, where they may be easily palpated as a
group. They may be differentiated just above the knee, the rectus
femoris being that portion of the muscle group just superior to the
patella, the vastus medialis forming the elevation above and medial to
the patella, and the vastus lateralis above and lateral to the patella.
The patellar ligament, the insertion of the four quadriceps muscles,
may be seen or easily palpated between the inferior border of the
patella and its insertion on the tibial tuberosity. Note the depressions
on either side of this ligament which are called the patellar depressions.
The upper part of the rectus femoris may be palpated near its origin
in the V-shaped space between the sartorius and the tensor fascia
latae. If you palpate about two inches below the anterior superior
iliac spine while your subject slightly flexes the hip, you will feel an
inverted V formed by the borders of these two muscles. As your subject extends the knee, you will feel the contraction of the rectus in this
space.

Medial Thigh

<u>HIP ADDUCTORS</u>

Position of Subject: Supine.
Bony Landmarks: Symphysis pubis and adductor tubercle.
Motions: Adduction with slight hip flexion and external rotation.
Resistance: Apply resistance on medial aspect of thigh just above
 knee, pulling thigh toward abduction.

Although it is difficult to differentiate between the two muscles, the
pectineus and adductor longus may be seen or easily palpated at the
upper part of the thigh just medial to the sartorius. The adductor
magnus may be palpated at its insertion on the adductor tubercle. The
gracilis is the most medial of the adductor muscles and will be most
easily identified later with the hamstring muscles.

Lateral Thigh

<u>GLUTEUS MEDIUS</u>

Position of Subject: Lying on side.
Skeletal Landmarks: Crest of ilium and greater trochanter.
Motions: Hip abduction with slight extension.
Resistance: Apply resistance on lateral side of thigh above knee, push-
 ing thigh toward adduction.

Palpate the muscle on the lateral aspect of the ilium, just posterior to
the tensor fascia latae. Trace it to its insertion on the greater
trochanter of the femur. Note that as the muscle contracts it causes a
depression just superior to the greater trochanter. This is referred
to as the lateral or gluteal depression. An alternate method of identifying the gluteus medius is to have your subject stand bearing all of his
weight on one leg. Palpate the muscle on the weight-bearing side.

Posterior Thigh

GLUTEUS MAXIMUS

Position of Subject: Prone.
Skeletal Landmark: Crest of ilium.
Motion: Hip extension and external rotation.
Resistance: Apply resistance just above knee, pushing thigh toward
  flexion.

The gluteus maximus may be easily palpated. It forms the contour of
the buttock.

HAMSTRINGS: SEMITENDINOSUS, SEMIMEMBRANOSUS, AND
BICEPS FEMORIS

Position of Subject: Prone.
Skeletal Landmarks: Ischial tuberosity, head of fibula, and medial
  condyle of tibia.
Motion: Knee flexion.
Resistance: Apply resistance just above ankle on posterior surface,
  pulling leg toward extension.

The semitendinosus and biceps femoris may be palpated as they
emerge from under the distal border of the gluteus maximus. They
form an elongated mass which is responsible for the contour of the
posterior thigh. The three hamstring muscles are best differentiated
and identified just superior to the knee. When these muscles contract
the popliteal space (the depression on the posterior surface of the knee)
becomes evident. The semitendinosus tendon may be easily seen and
palpated where it forms the medial border of the popliteal space. The
semimembranosus muscle is superficial only in the lower part of the
thigh where it forms a bulky mass which can be palpated on either side
of the semitendinosus tendon. The tendon of the gracilis, which is one
of the adductor muscles, may be palpated just medial to the semitendinosus tendon. It, like that of the semitendinosus, is a firm,
round tendon, but usually is slightly smaller. Asking your subject to
adduct the thigh as well may help in its identification. The tendon of
the biceps femoris may be easily seen and palpated where it forms the
lateral border of the popliteal space and may be traced to its insertion
on the head of the fibula. The common peroneal nerve may be palpated just superior and medial to the insertion of the biceps femoris.
Because of the superficial position of this nerve near the head of the

fibula, it is subject to injuries. For example, damage to the nerve may result from a short leg cast the upper border of which is too tight.

Anterior Leg

TIBIALIS ANTERIOR

Position of Subject: Supine.
Skeletal Landmarks: Lateral surface of tibia and base of first metatarsal.
Motions: Ankle dorsiflexion and inversion.
Resistance: Apply resistance on dorsal and medial surfaces of foot, pulling foot toward plantar flexion and eversion.

The muscle belly may be easily seen or palpated just lateral to the sharp anterior border of the tibia. Trace the large tendon, the most medial on the dorsum of the ankle, to its insertion on the base of the first metatarsal.

EXTENSOR HALLUCIS LONGUS

Position of Subject: Supine.
Skeletal Landmarks: Metatarsal and phalanges of great toe.
Motion: Extension of great toe.
Resistance: Apply resistance at distal end of great toe, pulling toe toward flexion.

The tendon may be seen or easily palpated on the dorsum of the ankle, just lateral to the tendon of the tibialis anterior. Trace it to its insertion on the great toe.

EXTENSOR DIGITORUM LONGUS

Position of Subject: Supine.
Skeletal Landmarks: Metatarsals of lateral four toes.
Motions: Extension of lateral four toes and dorsiflexion of ankle.
Resistance: Apply resistance to lateral four toes, pulling them toward flexion.

At the ankle the tendons may be seen or palpated as a group just lateral to the tendon of the extensor hallucis longus. As they cross the metatarsals they begin to separate and can be traced to their insertions on the lateral four toes.

PERONEUS TERTIUS

Position of Subject: Supine.
Skeletal Landmark: Base of fifth metatarsal.
Motions: Ankle dorsiflexion and eversion.
Resistance: Apply resistance at dorsal and lateral surfaces of foot, pushing foot toward plantar flexion and inversion.

The tendon, if present, may be palpated or seen on some subjects just lateral to the extensor digitorum longus tendon of the fifth toe. Trace it to its insertion on the base of the fifth metatarsal.

Lateral Leg

PERONEUS LONGUS AND BREVIS

Position of Subject: Supine.
Skeletal Landmarks: Fibula, lateral malleolus, and base of fifth metatarsal.
Motions: Ankle plantar flexion and eversion.
Resistance: Apply resistance at lateral and plantar surfaces of foot, pulling foot toward dorsiflexion and inversion.

The two muscle bellies may be palpated on the lateral side of the leg, along the anterolateral border of the fibula. As they contract you may see or easily palpate a depression which is called the lateral depression of the leg. The two tendons may be seen or palpated just posterior to the lateral malleolus. Follow the tendon of the peroneus longus to the cuboid bone where it enters the sole of the foot. Trace the peroneus brevis tendon along the lateral border of the foot to its insertion on the base of the fifth metatarsal.

Posterior Leg

GASTROCNEMIUS AND SOLEUS

Position of Subject: Standing.
Skeletal Landmark: Calcaneus.
Motion: Plantar flexion of ankle.
Resistance: Ask subject to stand on tiptoe. No added resistance is
   needed.

Both muscle bellies may be seen as they form the contour of the calf.
The gastrocnemius crosses the knee and is more bulky and superficial.
The soleus may be palpated or seen more easily at the lower part of
the leg where it emerges from under the gastrocnemius. Plantar
flexion of the ankle with the knees slightly flexed will cause a more
isolated contraction of the soleus. The tendons of these two muscles
plus that of the plantaris join to become the tendocalcaneus (Achilles
tendon), which may be easily seen or palpated superior to the posterior
border of the calcaneus.

TIBIALIS POSTERIOR

Position of Subject: Supine with foot extended over edge of table.
Skeletal Landmark: Medial malleolus.
Motions: Ankle plantar flexion and inversion.
Resistance: Apply resistance to plantar and medial surfaces of foot,
   pushing foot toward dorsiflexion and eversion.

The tendon may be palpated at the posterior aspect of and just superior
or inferior to the medial malleolus.

FLEXOR DIGITORUM LONGUS

Position of Subject: Supine with foot extended over edge of table.
Skeletal Landmark: Medial malleolus.
Motions: Ankle plantar flexion and flexion of lateral four toes.
Resistance: Apply resistance at plantar surface of foot and lateral four
   toes, pushing foot toward dorsiflexion and toes toward extension.

The tendon may be palpated at the posterior aspect of and just superior
or inferior to the medial malleolus, just lateral to the tendon of the
tibialis posterior. It is often difficult to differentiate between this
tendon and that of the tibialis posterior.

FLEXOR HALLUCIS LONGUS

Position of Subject: Supine with foot extended over edge of table.
Skeletal Landmark: Medial malleolus.
Motions: Ankle plantar flexion and flexion of great toe.
Resistance: Apply resistance to plantar surface of foot and great toe, pushing foot toward dorsiflexion and great toe toward extension.

The tendon may be palpated just medial and slightly deep to the tendocalcaneus.

Shoulder Girdle Motion

Motions of the shoulder girdle, the scapula, and the clavicle occur at the acromioclavicular and sternoclavicular joints. Although motion of the shoulder girdle is commonly referred to as scapular motion this is incorrect since the scapula and clavicle always move as a unit. Shoulder girdle motion is not as obvious as humeral motion, but is extremely important because movement of the upper extremity requires combined motions at the shoulder, glenohumeral joint, and at the two joints of the shoulder girdle.

TRANSLATORY OR LINEAR MOTION

During translatory motion the shoulder girdle moves as a whole and all parts move an equal distance. Note that when the shoulder girdle is abducted the vertebral border of the scapula is parallel to its location in the resting position. Abduction, adduction, elevation, and depression are translatory motions.

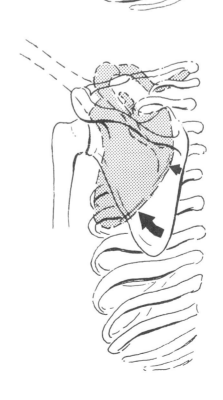

ROTATORY MOTION

During rotatory motion the shoulder girdle moves as a whole but all parts do not necessarily move an equal distance. Note that during upward rotation the inferior angle of the scapula has moved further than the medial angle. Upward and downward rotation are examples of rotatory motion.

Study the changing position of the scapula as the arm is moved.

1. Position your subject with his arms in a resting position at the sides of the body. With a skin pencil, outline the vertebral border and inferior angle of the scapula on your subject. The three drawings below represent the scapula in this position.

2. Ask your subject to flex his arm. Outline the vertebral border and inferior angle again. On the drawing labeled flexion super-impose a drawing of the scapula representing its changed position. If you have difficulty, palpation of the inferior angle of the scapula during the motion may be helpful.

3. Repeat this process with extension of the shoulder. On the drawing, superimpose a drawing of the scapula as it is positioned with the arm extended.

4. Repeat the process with the shoulder abducted.

5. Passive motion of the arm occurs only at the shoulder, gleno-humeral joint. To demonstrate this, ask your subject to completely relax the muscles of the shoulder girdle and arm. Passively move the arm into abduction and note that the resting position of the shoulder girdle is maintained.

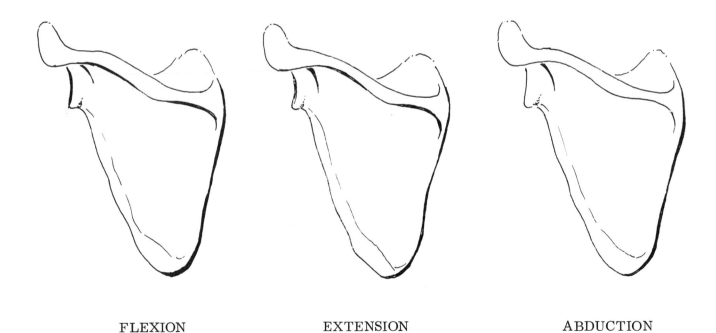

FLEXION   EXTENSION   ABDUCTION

Posterior Shoulder Girdle

TRAPEZIUS, UPPER

Position of Subject: Sitting.
Skeletal Landmarks: Occipital bone, cervical vertebrae, and
lateral aspect of the clavicle.
Motion: Shoulder girdle elevation.
Resistance: Apply resistance on superior surface of lateral aspect of
shoulder, pushing shoulder girdle down.

The muscle may be seen and easily palpated where it forms a triangle
between the clavicle, the occiput, and the cervical vertebrae. It is
responsible for the contour of the posterior shoulder and neck.

TRAPEZIUS, MIDDLE

Position of Subject: Prone, with arm in 90 degrees of abduction and
elbow flexed to 90 degrees. The upper arm should be supported on
the table with the forearm hanging over the edge.
Skeletal Landmarks: Vertebrae C_7 through T_4 and acromion process.
Motion: Shoulder girdle adduction. Ask your subject to lift his arm
off the table as far as possible.
Resistance: Apply resistance on posterior surface of lateral aspect of
shoulder, pushing shoulder girdle toward the table.

Palpate this portion of the muscle from the acromion medially to the
vertebrae.

TRAPEZIUS, LOWER

Position of Subject: Prone, with arm positioned straight overhead. The
arm should be resting on the table next to the head.
Skeletal Landmarks: Lower eight thoracic vertebrae and medial part of
scapular spine.
Motion: Scapular adduction and depression. Ask your subject to lift his
arm off the table, which will require the lower trapezius to stabilize
the scapula by pulling it down and in.
Resistance: No manual resistance is necessary.

Palpate this triangular portion of the muscle between the scapular
spine and the vertebrae and along the lower thoracic vertebrae.

RHOMBOIDS

Position of Subject: Prone with internal rotation of shoulder and elbow
  flexed. Ask your subject to put his hand on the lumbar area of his
  back.
Skeletal Landmarks: Lower cervical and upper thoracic vertebrae and
  vertebral border of scapula.
Motion: Shoulder girdle adduction and downward rotation. Ask your
  subject to lift his forearm and hand off his back.
Resistance: No manual resistance is necessary.

Using moderate pressure, palpate the muscle between the vertebrae
and the vertebral border of the scapula. The rhomboids are covered
by the trapezius which should be relaxed with the shoulder girdle in
this position.

LATISSIMUS DORSI AND TERES MAJOR

Position of Subject: Prone.
Skeletal Landmarks: Inferior angle of scapula, lateral aspect of ribs,
  and intertubercular groove of humerus.
Motion: Shoulder extension.
Resistance: Apply resistance just proximal to elbow joint, pushing
  arm toward flexion.

Palpate the bulky teres major between the inferior angle of the scapula
and the humerus. The flatter latissimus dorsi may be palpated just
inferior to the teres and on the posterolateral aspect of the ribs. These
two muscles make up the posterior wall of the axilla.

SERRATUS ANTERIOR

Position of Subject: Sitting with arm in 90 degrees of flexion, with
  elbow flexed. Ask your subject to touch his shoulder with his hand.
Skeletal Landmarks: Ribs, lateral side.
Motion: Shoulder girdle abduction and upward rotation. Ask your subject to thrust his elbow forward. Do not allow him to substitute by
  flexing the trunk.
Resistance: Apply resistance at point of elbow, pushing arm in
  posterior direction.

The lower part of this muscle may be palpated near its origin on the
lateral aspect of ribs 5, 6, 7, and 8, just anterior to the latissimus
dorsi. Palpate on the lateral aspect of the ribs at the level of the lower
part of the scapula.

POSTERIOR DELTOID

Position of Subject: Prone with arm in 90 degrees of abduction and
  elbow flexed to 90 degrees. The upper arm should be supported on
  the table with the forearm hanging over the edge.
Skeletal Landmarks: Lateral part of scapular spine and lateral aspect
  of humerus.
Motion: Shoulder horizontal abduction.
Resistance: Apply resistance just proximal to elbow joint, pushing arm
  toward horizontal adduction.

The posterior fibers of the deltoid may be seen and easily palpated
from origin to insertion.

INFRASPINATUS AND TERES MINOR

Position of Subject: Prone, with arm in 90 degrees of abduction and
  with elbow flexed to 90 degrees. The upper arm should be supported
  on the table with the forearm hanging over the edge.
Skeletal Landmark: Lateral border of scapula.
Motion: Shoulder external rotation.
Resistance: Apply resistance just proximal to wrist joint, pushing arm
  toward internal rotation.

The two muscles may be palpated near the lateral border of the scapula,
between the posterior deltoid and the teres major. Although it may be
difficult to differentiate between the two muscles on a normal subject,
the infraspinatus is immediately inferior to the deltoid and the teres
minor is just superior to the teres major.

Anterior Shoulder Girdle

PECTORALIS MAJOR

Position of Subject: Supine.
Skeletal Landmarks: Anterior aspect of upper ribs, medial part of
  clavicle, and intertubercular groove of humerus.
Motion: Horizontal adduction.
Resistance: Apply resistance just proximal to elbow joint, pulling
  arm toward horizontal abduction.

Both heads of the pectoralis major will be seen contracting and may be easily palpated. Note that the lateral portion of the muscle, between the rib cage and the humerus, forms the anterior wall of the axilla. The clavicular head may be easily differentiated from the sternal head by the following method. With your subject seated and the arm in approximately 90 degrees of flexion, alternately apply resistance to flexion and extension of the shoulder. (Place your hands above and below the subject's arm and ask him to alternately push up against one hand and down against the other hand.)

ANTERIOR DELTOID

Position of Subject: Supine or sitting.
Skeletal Landmarks: Lateral part of clavicle and lateral aspect of
   humerus.
Motion: Shoulder flexion to 90 degrees.
Resistance: Apply resistance just proximal to elbow, pushing arm
   toward extension.

The anterior deltoid may be easily seen and palpated from its origin on the clavicle to its insertion on the humerus. Notice that the clavicular head of the pectoralis major is also contracting during this motion. A triangular-shaped depression, the infraclavicular fossa, separates these two muscles at their origin.

MIDDLE DELTOID

Position of Subject: Supine or sitting.
Skeletal Landmarks: Acromion process of scapula and humerus.
Motion: Shoulder abduction to 90 degrees.
Resistance: Apply resistance just proximal to elbow, pushing arm
   toward adduction.

The muscle may be seen and easily palpated on the most lateral aspect of the shoulder.

Anterior Arm, Forearm, and Hand

BICEPS BRACHII

Position of Subject: Sitting, with arm at side and forearm supinated.
Motion: Elbow flexion to 90 degrees.
Resistance: Apply resistance just proximal to wrist joint, pushing
   forearm toward extension.

The muscle belly is easily seen since it forms the contour of the
anterior arm. The tendon may be palpated on the antecubital fossa,
the depression on the anterior surface of the elbow joint. The flat,
fan-shaped, lacertus fibrosis may be identified just medial to the tendon where it becomes continuous with the deep fascia.

BRACHIORADIALIS

Position of Subject: Sitting with arm at side and forearm in mid-
   position between pronation and supination.
Skeletal Landmark: Lateral supracondylar ridge of humerus.
Motion: Elbow flexion to 90 degrees.
Resistance: Apply resistance just proximal to wrist, pushing forearm
   toward extension.

The muscle may be seen and easily palpated from the lower lateral
aspect of the humerus to the middle of the forearm. The upper part
of the muscle forms the lateral border of the antecubital fossa.

PRONATOR TERES

Position of Subject: Sitting with elbow flexed to 90 degrees and forearm
   supinated.
Skeletal Landmark: Medial epicondyle of humerus.
Motion: Forearm pronation.
Resistance: Apply resistance proximal to wrist, turning forearm
   toward supination.

The muscle may be seen or easily palpated from the medial epicondyle
of the humerus to the medial border of the brachioradialis muscle.
This muscle forms the medial border of the antecubital fossa.

FLEXOR CARPI ULNARIS, PALMARIS LONGUS, AND FLEXOR CARPI RADIALIS

Position of Subject: Sitting with forearm
 supinated.
Skeletal Landmarks: Distal part of radius
 and ulna and pisiform.
Motion: Wrist flexion.

The bellies of these muscles, along with the
flexor digitorum superficialis, may be palpated as a group just medial to the pronator
teres. These four muscles have a common
origin from the medial epicondyle, called
the common flexor tendon. They may be
differentiated at the wrist where the tendons are easily palpated. Palpate the tendon
of the flexor carpi ulnaris at the medial side
of the wrist and follow it to its attachment on
the pisiform. The tendon will also become
prominent when abduction of the fifth finger
is resisted. The palmaris longus tendon, if
present, may be easily seen at the center of
the wrist. The flexor carpi radialis tendon
may be seen or palpated about one fourth of
an inch lateral to the tendon of the palmaris
longus. Also, locate the radial artery just
lateral to the flexor carpi radialis tendon by
palpating for the pulse beat.

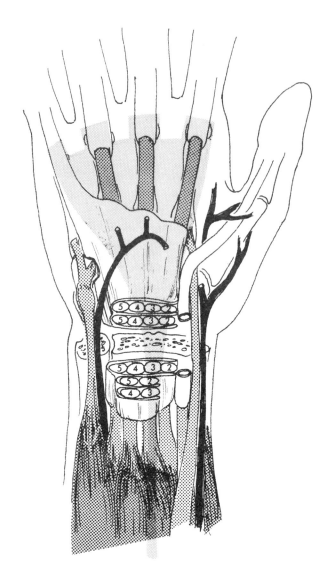

FLEXOR DIGITORUM SUPERFICIALIS

Position of Subject: Sitting with forearm supinated and wrist slightly
 flexed.
Motions: Flexion of proximal interphalangeal joints of four fingers.
Resistance: Apply resistance on body of middle phalanx, pushing
 fingers toward extension.

Palpate the tendons at the wrist on either side of and deep to the tendon
of the palmaris longus. The two most superficial of the four tendons
are those which attach to the third and fourth fingers.

ABDUCTOR POLLICIS BREVIS

Position of Subject: Sitting with dorsum of hand resting on table and thumb adducted. The ulnar side of the thumb should be touching the palm of the hand.
Skeletal Landmark: First metacarpal.
Motion: Abduction of thumb. Ask your subject to raise the thumb off the palm of the hand — the motion will be perpendicular to the palm of the hand.
Resistance: Apply resistance on lateral side of first phalanx, pushing thumb toward adduction.

The muscle belly may be seen and palpated on the lateral surface of the first metacarpal.

FLEXOR POLLICIS BREVIS

Position of Subject: Sitting with dorsum of hand resting on table.
Skeletal Landmark: First metacarpal.
Motion: Flexion at metacarpophalangeal joint of thumb.
Resistance: Apply resistance on anterior surface of proximal phalanx, pushing thumb toward extension.

The muscle may be seen or palpated on the anterior surface of the first metacarpal.

ADDUCTOR POLLICIS

Position of Subject: Sitting with dorsum of hand resting on table.
Skeletal Landmark: First metacarpal.
Motion: Thumb adduction.
Resistance: Apply resistance at head of first metacarpal, pulling thumb toward abduction.

The muscle may be palpated in a triangular space between the first dorsal interosseous and the medial margin of the thenar eminence.

FLEXOR DIGITI MINIMI

Position of Subject: Sitting with dorsum of hand resting on table.
Skeletal Landmark: Fifth metacarpal.
Motion: Flexion at metacarpophalangeal joint of fifth finger.
Resistance: Apply resistance on volar surface of proximal phalanx, pushing finger toward extension.

Palpate the muscle on the anterior surface of the fifth metacarpal.

Position of Subject: Sitting with dorsum of hand resting on table.
Skeletal Landmark: Fifth metacarpal.
Motion: Abduction of fifth finger.
Resistance: Apply resistance on medial side of proximal phalanx, pushing finger toward adduction.

Palpate the muscle on the medial side of the fifth metacarpal.

Posterior Arm

TRICEPS

Position of Subject: Prone with arm abducted to 90 degrees, elbow flexed, and forearm hanging over edge of table.
Skeletal Landmarks: Posterior aspect of humerus and olecranon process.
Motion: Elbow extension.
Resistance: Apply resistance just proximal to wrist, pushing forearm toward flexion.

The flat tendon of insertion of the triceps is easily palpated where it attaches to the olecranon process. The long head may be identified on the medial side of the posterior arm as it emerges from the inferior border of the posterior deltoid. The lateral head may be palpated on the posterolateral surface of the arm. The medial head is most easily identified on the lower portion of the posteromedial surface of the arm, superior to the medial epicondyle.

Posterior Forearm and Hand

Remembering the location of the tendons as they cross the wrist joint is important for understanding muscle action on that joint. On the illustration showing a cross section of the wrist the tunnels through which the tendons pass are numbered. The muscles will be listed below as their tendons appear in the tunnels from the radial side, tunnel 1, to the ulnar side, tunnel 6.

ABDUCTOR POLLICIS LONGUS (1)

Position of Subject: Sitting with medial side
   of hand resting on table.
Skeletal Landmark: Base of first metacarpal.
Motion: Extension and abduction of thumb.
Resistance: Apply resistance at distal end of
   first metacarpal, pushing thumb toward
   little finger.

The tendon may be palpated just proximal to
the first metacarpal at the most lateral
aspect of the wrist.

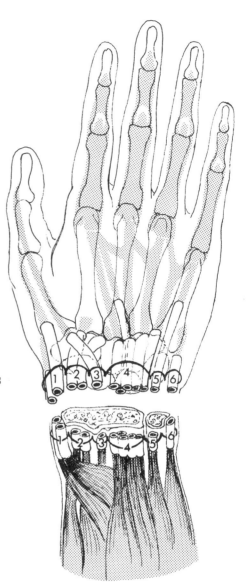

EXTENSOR POLLICIS BREVIS (1)

Position of Subject: Sitting with medial side
   of hand resting on table.
Skeletal Landmarks: Styloid process of radius
   and base of proximal phalanx of thumb.
Resistance: Apply resistance at distal end of
   proximal phalanx, pushing proximal phalanx
   toward flexion.

The tendon may be seen or palpated next to
that of the abductor pollicis longus and may
be traced from the radial styloid process to
the base of the proximal phalanx.

EXTENSOR CARPI RADIALIS LONGUS AND BREVIS (2)

Position of Subject: Sitting with palmar surface of hand resting on table.
Skeletal Landmarks: Lateral epicondyle of humerus and bases of second
   and third metacarpals.
Resistance: Apply resistance at distal end of metacarpals, pushing
   hand toward flexion.

The bellies of these two muscles may be palpated in the area between
the lateral epicondyle of the humerus and the middle of the dorsum of
the forearm. Palpate the tendon of the extensor carpi radialis longus
at its insertion on the base of the second metacarpal. The tendon of
the extensor carpi radialis brevis will be found on the ulnar side of the
extensor carpi radialis longus tendon, proximal to the base of the third
metacarpal.

EXTENSOR POLLICIS LONGUS (3)

Position of Subject: Sitting with medial side of hand resting on table.
Skeletal Landmarks: Tubercle of Lister and base of distal phalanx of
    thumb.
Motion: Thumb extension.
Resistance: Apply resistance on dorsum of distal phalanx, pushing
    thumb toward flexion.

The tendon may be traced from the tubercle of Lister to the base of
the distal phalanx. The tendons of the two thumb extensors form the
borders of a depression known as the anatomic snuffbox.

EXTENSOR DIGITORUM (4), EXTENSOR INDICIS (4), AND EXTENSOR DIGITI MINIMI (5)

Position of Subject: Sitting with palmar surface of hand resting on
    table.
Skeletal Landmarks: Dorsal surface of metacarpals.
Motion: Extension of four fingers.
Resistance: Apply resistance on dorsal surface of proximal
    phalanges, pushing four phalanges toward flexion.

The muscle belly of the extensor digitorum may be palpated on the
dorsum of the forearm, medial to that of the extensor carpi radialis
brevis. Palpate the tendons of the extensor digitorum and the extensor
indicis as a group at the center of the wrist. At the wrist, the
extensor digiti minimi tendon will be found on the ulnar side of the
extensor digitorum tendons. On the dorsum of the hand the tendons of
the extensor digitorum may be traced to each of the four fingers. The
tendon of the extensor digitorum to the fifth finger is smaller than the
others and can best be palpated just proximal to the metacarpophalangeal joints of the fourth and fifth fingers. The tendon of the
extensor indicis will be found deep to and slightly medial to the extensor
digitorum tendon to the index finger. The tendon of the extensor digiti
minimi may be easily palpated on the dorsal surface of the fifth metacarpal.

EXTENSOR CARPI ULNARIS (6)

Position of Subject: Sitting with palmar surface of hand resting on
table.
Skeletal Landmarks: Head of ulna and base of fifth metacarpal.
Motion: Wrist extension.
Resistance: Apply resistance on dorsum of metacarpals, pushing hand
toward flexion.

The tendon is the most medial on the dorsum of the wrist and may be
palpated between the head of the ulna and the base of the fifth metacarpal.

DORSAL INTEROSSEI

Position of Subject: Sitting with palmar surface of hand resting on
table.
Skeletal Landmarks: Metacarpals.
Motion: Abduction of index, middle, and ring fingers.
Resistance: Apply resistance on radial side of index finger, on both
sides of middle finger, and on ulnar side of ring finger, pushing
each finger toward adduction. Remember that the axis for abduction-
adduction runs down the center of the middle finger; therefore, motion
in either direction of that finger is abduction.

The first dorsal interosseous may be seen or easily palpated on the
radial side of the second metacarpal. The dorsal interossei to the
middle and ring fingers may be palpated on the dorsum of the hand,
between the metacarpals.

Kinesiology

Introduction

Kinesiology is the study of human movement. Such study requires knowledge of the anatomy of the skeletal and neuromuscular systems, consideration of the mechanical factors which affect motion, and analysis of the ways in which muscles act together to provide coordinated movement. This section of the manual was designed to guide your analysis of each of the motions possible at each of the joints of the human body.

Although the movements which we use in everyday life are complex, combinations of motion usually involving several joints, their study requires precise definition with an axis for motion designated. Therefore, the motions presented in this section are oriented to the three planes of the body, the sagittal, the coronal, and the horizontal. Each motion occurs around an axis which is perpendicular to the plane of motion. The planes and axes are presented for the purpose of defining the motions to be studied.

Motions in a Sagittal Plane around a Coronal Axis

Shoulder: Flexion and extension
Elbow: Flexion and extension
Wrist: Flexion and extension
Fingers: Flexion and extension
Hip: Flexion and extension
Knee: Flexion and extension
Ankle: Dorsi and plantar flexion
Thumb: Abduction

Motions in a Coronal Plane around a Sagittal Axis

Shoulder: Abduction and adduction
Wrist: Radial and ulnar deviation
Thumb: Extension
Hip: Abduction and adduction
Foot: Eversion and inversion

Motions in a Horizontal Plane around a Vertical Axis

Shoulder: Internal and external rotation
Forearm: Supination and pronation
Hip: Internal and external rotation

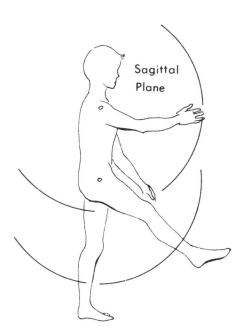 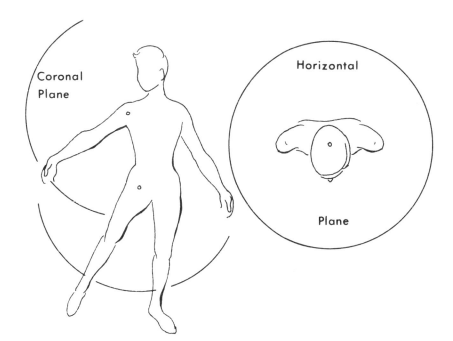

Place the point of a toothpick on either dot. It represents the coronal axis. The arm and thigh flex and extend in a sagittal plane.

Holding the toothpick on these dots demonstrates the sagittal axis. Abduction and adduction occur in the coronal plane.

In this example the toothpick represents the vertical axis. Rotation of the head, arm, leg, or trunk occurs in the horizontal plane.

The illustrations in this section were designed to depict the functional and mechanical aspects of the musculoskeletal system rather than the precise anatomic features. On each drawing you will find the axis for motion designated by a circle or a rod. Zip-A-Tone Screen patterns are used in an attempt to show the layers of muscles on a single illustration and also to show the relationship of each muscle to the group of muscles. Labeling of the muscles was purposely omitted since we believe that greater learning will be achieved if you must identify each muscle as you study the group.

The text for each motion lists the muscles which perform the action being considered. Each is either a prime mover or an accessory. The name of each prime mover is underlined and its attachments and innervation are given. We have used the symbol O to designate the origin, I to designate insertion, and N to designate innervation. This designation was chosen only for ease of presentation. It is in no way intended to suggest that the origin is the fixed point and that the action occurs at the insertion. To avoid this concept the use of proximal and distal attachment is preferred by many kinesiologists. The amount of detail included in the description of muscle attachments has been limited to that which seems most important for understanding function. More detailed descriptions may be found in most standard anatomy textbooks. The muscles that may act as accessories for the action are also listed. Their attachments and innervation are given under the action or actions which they perform as prime movers. In parentheses after the name of each muscle is a listing of the other actions it is capable of performing.

To maximize your learning the utilization of a skeleton to augment the information in the manual is recommended. Simulation of a muscle may be achieved by placing one end of a strip of gauze on the proximal attachment and the other end on the distal attachment. The gauze will fairly accurately designate the line of action of the muscle which then can be considered in relation to the axis or axes of motion of the joint.

The following procedure is suggested for your analysis of each motion:

1. Analyze each muscle listed, both prime movers and accessories. Read the description of the attachments, locate the points of attachment on the illustration, and identify the muscle. Locate the axis for motion. Simulate the muscle on the skeleton with a gauze strip. Look at the line of pull of the muscle, consider its relationship to the axis for motion, and determine why it is capable of performing the motion being studied. This method of analysis will facilitate the learning of muscle attachments. It is also important to remember that as the total range of motion occurs, the ability of an individual muscle to perform the motion may change owing to mechanical and/or physiological factors. Consequently, you should move the extremity to different positions within the range of motion and consider how the line of pull of each muscle has changed in relation to the axis for motion.

2. Study the muscle group to determine how the muscles act together in the performance of the motion. If a muscle contracts in isolation it will perform all the actions it is capable of performing. If

the desired motion is just one of its actions, some other force, usually the contraction of another muscle, must rule out or neutralize the undesired actions. For example, if the desired motion at the wrist is flexion, the flexor carpi ulnaris and flexor carpi radialis must contract together. If the flexor carpi ulnaris contracts alone, it will flex and ulnarly deviate. If the flexor carpi radialis contracts alone, it will flex with deviation in a radial direction. When they contract together the radial and ulnar deviation actions are neutralized and flexion occurs. In this manual this is referred to as the synergistic action of muscles. Consider the other actions of each muscle — those listed in parentheses after the muscle name. Are there other muscles within the group which can act synergistically to neutralize the undesired motion or is it necessary for some other muscle group to function in this capacity?

3. Determine the fixating forces required for effective action of the muscle group. Usually muscles are equally capable of moving either skeletal segment to which they are attached and if allowed to do so will move both bones simultaneously. If the muscles are to apply their force efficiently to move just one of the skeletal segments, the other bone to which they are attached must be fixated or stabilized. For example, the muscles which flex the hip are equally capable of moving the femur or moving the pelvis. If movement of the femur is desired, some other force, in this case contraction of the abdominal muscles, must prevent the pelvic motion. Muscles which act in this way to stabilize one bony segment will be called fixators in this manual. Although we tend to think of muscles primarily as movers their function as stabilizers or fixators is often of equal or greater importance.

4. If the proximal attachment of a group of prime movers such as the hip flexors is fixated what motion will occur? Muscles are generally classified according to the actions they perform when their contracting force is applied to their distal attachment. For example, the iliopsoas muscle is classified as a hip flexor. As previously stated, muscles are equally capable of applying their force at the proximal attachment and this type of function is frequently required of some muscles. When you come to a sitting position from a back lying position most of the motion occurs at the hip joint. In this case the hip flexors are applying their force at their proximal attachment to move the pelvis.

Your analysis up to this point has been related to the actions performed by muscles when they contract concentrically, a shortening contraction. To appreciate completely the musculoskeletal system and the complex actions required of muscles to achieve even the simple motor activities we so readily take for granted, you must study the other ways in which muscles function. Muscles are also required to contract eccentrically and isometrically. The eccentric contraction, a lengthening contraction, is commonly required to control a motion. For example, if gravity provides the force for a movement, an eccentric contraction of muscles is required to control, or brake, the motion. If you bend down to pick up an object from the floor, gravity provides the force for the movement and the back and hip extensor muscles must contract eccentrically to control the motion. Muscles are also required to contract without a change in length, an isometric contraction, to maintain the position of a skeletal segment. In some instances both the agonist and antagonist muscles must contract to maintain a joint in a stable position. This is called cocontraction of muscles. As you analyze activities you must always determine what force is causing the motion and the type of contraction of each muscle group that is acting.

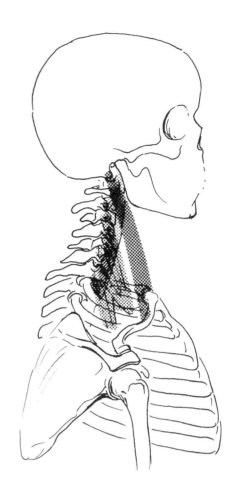

Neck Flexion

STERNOCLEIDOMASTOID (Neck rotation)

O: Superior border of the sternum and medial part of the clavicle.
I: Mastoid process.
N: Spinal accessory and C_2 and C_3.

LONGUS COLLI AND LONGUS CAPITIS

O: Lower cervical and upper thoracic vertebrae, anterior surfaces.
I: Upper cervical vertebrae, anterior surfaces, and occipital bone.
N: Adjacent spinal nerves.

Accessory Muscle:
SCALENE MUSCLES (Neck rotation)
O: Cervical vertebrae, transverse processes.
I: First and second ribs, anterolateral surface.
N: Adjacent spinal nerves.

Lateral Flexion

Lateral flexion of the neck is performed by the unilateral contraction
of the neck flexors and neck extensors with motion occurring in a
coronal plane.

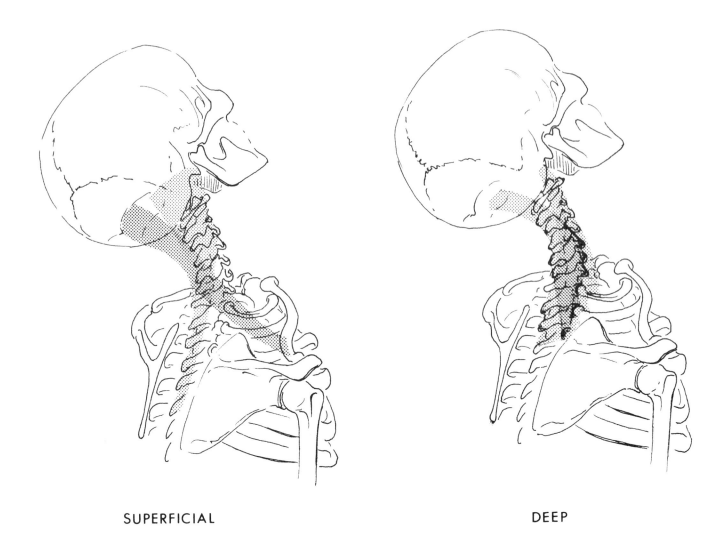

SUPERFICIAL

DEEP

Neck Extension

TRAPEZIUS, UPPER (Neck rotation; shoulder girdle elevation, upward
   rotation and adduction)

O: Occipital protuberance and ligamentum nuchae.
I: Clavicle, superior surface of the lateral part.
N: Spinal accessory and C_3 and C_4.

SPLENIUS CAPITIS AND CERVICIS (Neck rotation)

O: Lower ligamentum nuchae and spinous processes of the upper
   thoracic vertebrae.
I: Mastoid process, occipital bone, upper cervical vertebrae,
   transverse processes.
N: Spinal nerves, dorsal branches.

SEMISPINALIS CAPITIS AND CERVICIS (Neck rotation)

O: Upper thoracic and lower cervical vertebrae transverse processes.
I: Upper cervical vertebrae spinous processes and occipital bone.
N: Spinal nerves, dorsal branches.

ERECTOR SPINAE GROUP, CERVICIS AND CAPITIS DIVISIONS

O: Lower cervical, upper thoracic vertebrae transverse processes,
   and spinous processes and upper ribs.
I: Upper cervical vertebrae and occipital bone.
N: Spinal nerves, dorsal branches.

Accessory Muscles:
TRANSVERSOSPINALIS MUSCLE GROUP (Neck rotation)
LEVATOR SCAPULAE

Neck Rotation

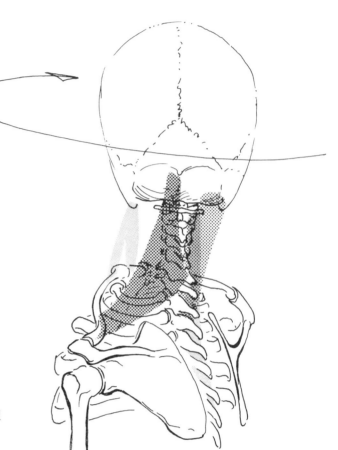

Rotation to the Right

LEFT STERNOCLEIDOMASTOID
(Neck flexion)

O: Superior border of the sternum and
medial part of the clavicle.
I: Mastoid process.
N: Spinal accessory and C_2 and C_3.

LEFT TRAPEZIUS, UPPER (Neck extension; shoulder girdle elevation,
adduction and upward rotation)

O: Occipital protuberance and ligamentum nuchae.
I: Clavicle, superior surface of lateral part.
N: Spinal accessory and C_3 and C_4.

RIGHT SPLENIUS CAPITIS AND CERVICIS (Neck extension)

O: Lower ligamentum nuchae and spinous processes of the upper
thoracic vertebrae.
I: Mastoid process and occipital bone.
N: Spinal nerves, dorsal branches.

Accessory Muscles:
LEFT SCALENES (Neck flexion)
LEFT TRANSVERSOSPINALIS GROUP (Neck extension)

Rotation to the Left

The opposite muscles will contract.

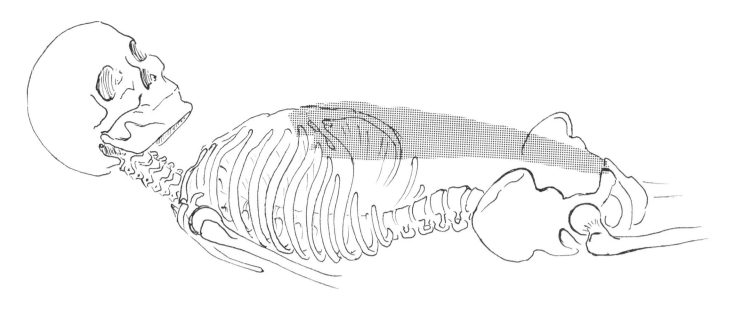

Trunk Forward Flexion

<u>RECTUS ABDOMINIS</u>

O: Crest of the pubis.
I: Inferior border of the sternum and costal cartilages of ribs 5, 6, and 7.
N: Lower intercostals.

Accessory Muscles:
EXTERNAL OBLIQUE ABDOMINIS (Trunk rotation)
INTERNAL OBLIQUE ABDOMINIS (Trunk rotation)

Lateral Flexion

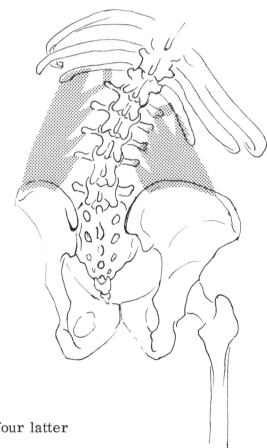

<u>QUADRATUS LUMBORUM</u> (Trunk extension)

O: Posterior iliac crest and transverse processes of the lower lumbar vertebrae.
I: Twelfth rib, transverse processes of the upper lumbar vertebrae.
N: T_{12}, L_1, L_2.

<u>INTERNAL OBLIQUE ABDOMINIS</u> (Trunk rotation)

<u>EXTERNAL OBLIQUE ABDOMINIS</u> (Trunk rotation)

<u>ERECTOR SPINAE GROUP</u> (Trunk extension)

<u>TRANSVERSOSPINALIS GROUP</u> (Trunk extension)

Note: For origins, insertions, and innervations of the four latter muscles, see the next two pages.

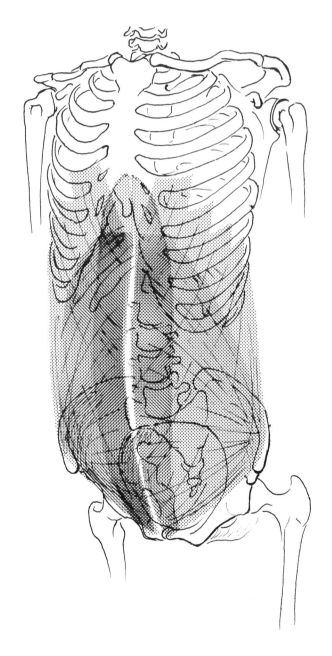

ABDOMINAL MUSCLES

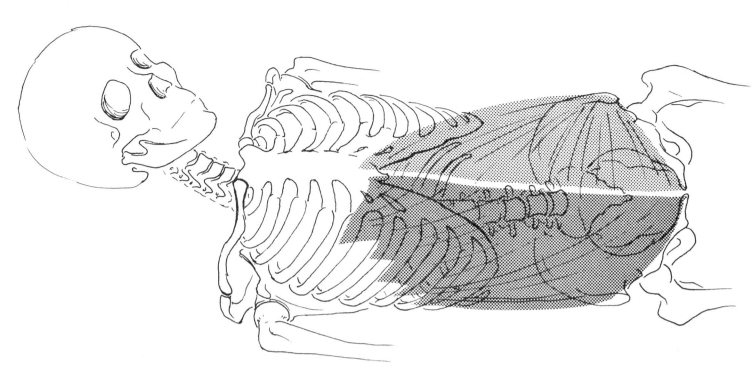

Trunk Flexion with Rotation

Rotation to the Left

LEFT INTERNAL OBLIQUE ABDOMINIS

O: Anterior iliac crest, lateral inguinal ligament, lumbodorsal fascia.
I: Costal cartilages of the lower ribs, linea alba, and pubis.
N: Lower intercostals, iliohypogastric, and ilioinguinal.

RIGHT EXTERNAL OBLIQUE ABDOMINIS

O: Lower eight ribs, anterolateral aspect.
I: Anterior iliac crest and linea alba.
N: Lower intercostals, iliohypogastric, and ilioinguinal.

Rotation to the Right

The right internal oblique and the left external oblique muscles contract.

Note: When the trunk is rotated without flexion the erector spinae and the transversospinalis muscle groups also function. The transversus abdominis, the deepest of the abdominal muscle group, does not contribute to trunk motions. Along with the other muscles, its function is to support and compress the abdomen.

Trunk Extension

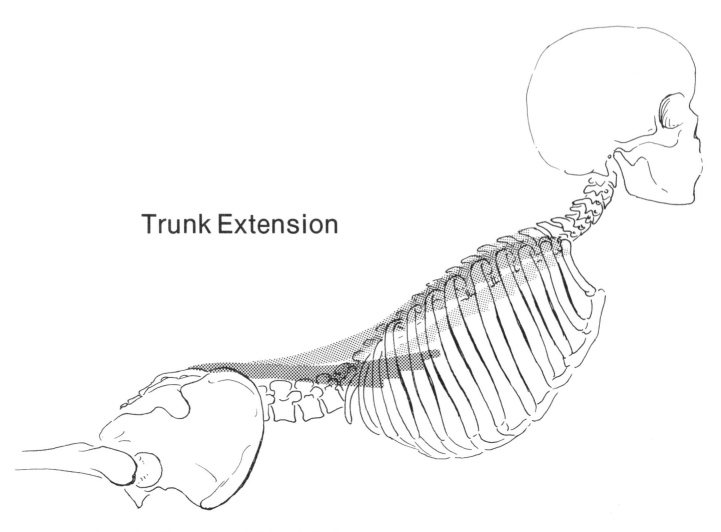

Erector Spinae Group (Trunk lateral flexion):

ILIOCOSTALIS LUMBORUM

O: Sacrum, lower thoracic and lumbar vertebrae, posterior iliac
    crests.
I: Angles of the lower ribs.
N: Spinal nerves, dorsal branches.

ILIOCOSTALIS THORACIS

O: Lower ribs, posterior surfaces.
I: Upper ribs, posterior surfaces.
N: Spinal nerves, dorsal branches.

LONGISSIMUS THORACIS

O: Lumbar vertebrae and lumbodorsal fascia.
I: All thoracic vertebrae and ribs.
N: Spinal nerves, dorsal branches.

SPINALIS THORACIS

O: Lower thoracic and upper lumbar vertebrae.
I: Upper thoracic vertebrae.
N: Spinal nerves, dorsal branches.

Transversospinalis Muscle Group
(Trunk lateral flexion):

SEMISPINALIS
MULTIFIDI
INTERSPINALIS
ROTATORS
INTERTRANSVERSARI

The specific origins and insertions of
each of these muscles are not given
since they function as a group. All
originate on vertebrae and insert on
higher vertebrae, spanning from one
to several vertebral segments. The
direction of their fibers is medial and
all are innervated by dorsal branches
of spinal nerves.

Accessory Muscle:
QUADRATUS LUMBORUM

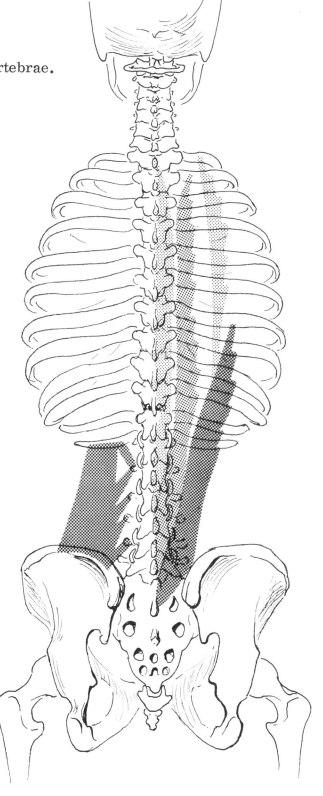

DEEP BACK MUSCLES

53

Hip Flexion

ILIOPSOAS, Psoas Major and Iliacus

O: Iliac fossa, sides of the twelfth thoracic and all of the lumbar vertebrae.
I: Femur, lesser trochanter.
N: Psoas — L_2-L_3, iliacus — femoral.

SARTORIUS (Hip abduction and external rotation; knee flexion; knee medial rotation)

O: Anterior superior iliac spine.
I: Tibia, anterior surface of the medial condyle.
N: Femoral.

RECTUS FEMORIS (Knee extension)

O: Straight head — anterior inferior iliac spine. Reflected head — superior rim of the acetabulum.
I: Patella and tibial tuberosity via the patellar ligament.
N: Femoral.

Accessory Muscles:
TENSOR FASCIA LATAE (Hip abduction and internal rotation; knee lateral rotation)
PECTINEUS (Hip adduction)
ADDUCTOR BREVIS AND LONGUS (Hip adduction)
ADDUCTOR MAGNUS, OBLIQUE FIBERS (Hip adduction)
GLUTEUS MEDIUS, ANTERIOR FIBERS (Hip abduction and internal rotation)
GLUTEUS MINIMUS (Hip abduction and internal rotation)

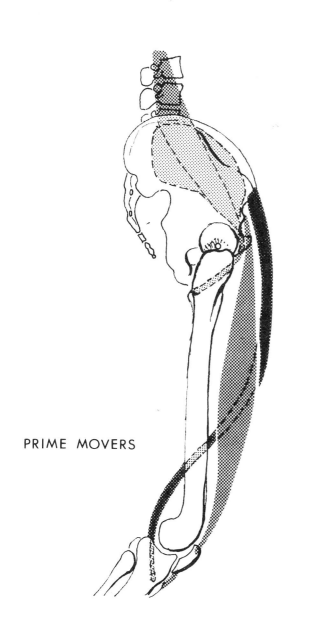

PRIME MOVERS

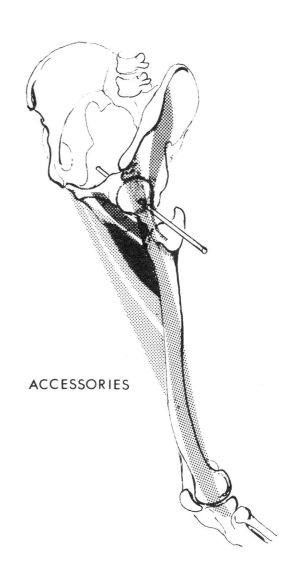

ACCESSORIES

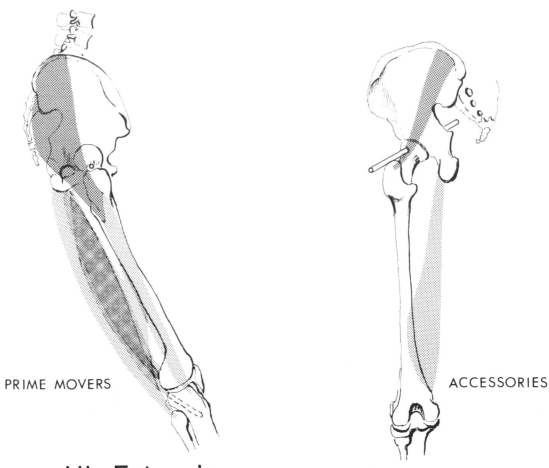

PRIME MOVERS   ACCESSORIES

Hip Extension

GLUTEUS MAXIMUS (Hip external rotation)

O: Iliac crest and posterior gluteal line, lateral border of the sacrum.
I: Superficial fibers — iliotibial band.
N: Inferior gluteal.

HAMSTRINGS (Knee flexion; knee rotation)

O: SEMIMEMBRANOSUS, SEMITENDINOSUS, BICEPS, LONG HEAD — ischial tuberosity.
I: SEMIMEMBRANOSUS — tibia, posterior surface of the medial condyle. SEMITENDINOSUS — tibia, anterior surface of the medial condyle. BICEPS FEMORIS — head of fibula, lateral aspect.
N: Sciatic, tibial division.

Accessory Muscles:
GLUTEUS MEDIUS, POSTERIOR FIBERS (Hip abduction and external rotation)
ADDUCTOR MAGNUS, VERTICAL FIBERS (Hip adduction and internal rotation)

56

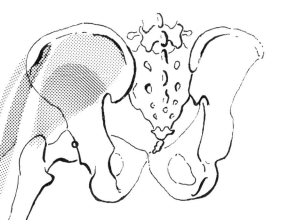

Hip Abduction

GLUTEUS MEDIUS (Anterior fibers — hip flexion and internal rotation; posterior fibers — hip extension and external rotation)

O: Ilium, crest and area between the anterior and the posterior gluteal lines.
I: Femur, lateral aspect of the greater trochanter.
N: Superior gluteal.

GLUTEUS MINIMUS (Hip flexion and internal rotation)

O: Ilium, area between the anterior and the inferior gluteal lines.
I: Femur, anterior aspect of the greater trochanter.
N: Superior gluteal.

TENSOR FASCIA LATAE (Hip flexion and internal rotation; knee lateral rotation)

O: Iliac crest, anterior part of the outer surface.
I: Iliotibial band, which attaches to the anterior aspect of the lateral tibial condyle.
N: Superior gluteal.

Accessory Muscle:
SARTORIUS (Hip flexion and external rotation; knee flexion; knee medial rotation)

Hip Adduction

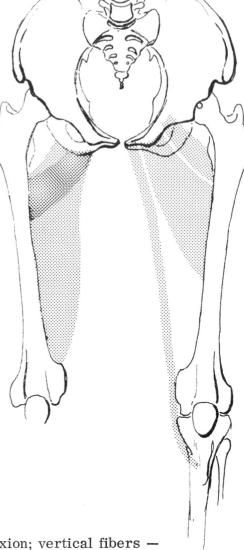

DEEP

SUPERFICIAL

<u>PECTINEUS</u> (Hip flexion)

O: Pubic pectin.
I: Femur, pectineal line.
N: Femoral or obturator.

<u>ADDUCTOR BREVIS</u> (Hip flexion)

O: Pubis, inferior ramus.
I: Femur, superior part of the linea aspera.
N: Obturator.

<u>ADDUCTOR LONGUS</u> (Hip flexion)

O: Pubis, superior ramus.
I: Femur, middle part of the linea aspera.
N: Obturator.

<u>ADDUCTOR MAGNUS</u> (Oblique fibers — hip flexion; vertical fibers — hip extension and internal rotation)

O: Oblique fibers — inferior rami of the pubis and ischium; vertical fibers — ischial tuberosity.
I: Oblique fibers — femur, superior part of the linea aspera; vertical fibers — femur, inferior part of the linea aspera, and the adductor tubercle.
N: Oblique fibers — obturator; vertical fibers — sciatic, tibial division.

<u>GRACILIS</u> (Knee flexion; knee medial rotation)

O: Pubis, inferior ramus.
I: Tibia, anterior surface of the medial condyle.
N: Obturator.

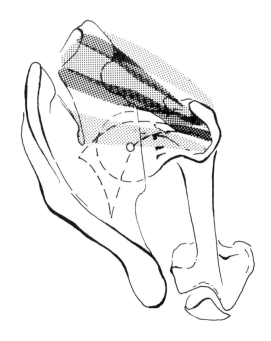

LEFT PELVIS AND FEMUR : SUPERIOR VIEW

Hip External Rotation

OBTURATOR INTERNUS

O: Inner margin of the obturator foramen and membrane.
I: Femur, inner surface of the greater trochanter.
N: L_5, S_1, S_2.

OBTURATOR EXTERNUS

O: External margin of the obturator foramen and membrane.
I: Femur, inner surface of the greater trochanter.
N: Obturator.

GEMELLI

O: Superior — ischium, superior aspect of the lesser sciatic notch;
   inferior — ischium, inferior aspect of the lesser sciatic notch.
I: Femur, inner surface of the greater trochanter via the obturator
   internus tendon.
N: Superior — nerve to the obturator internus; inferior — nerve to the
   quadratus femoris.

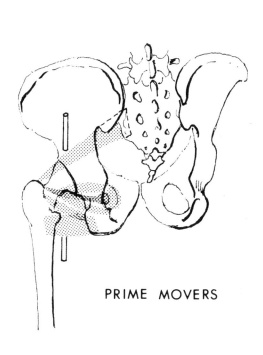

PRIME MOVERS

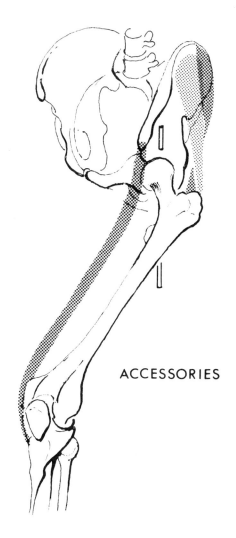

ACCESSORIES

QUADRATUS FEMORIS

O: Ischial tuberosity, superior aspect.
I: Femur, greater trochanter, inferior aspect.
N: L_4, L_5, S_1.

PIRIFORMIS

O: Second, third, and fourth sacral vertebrae, anterior surface.
I: Femur, inner surface of the greater trochanter.
N: S_2, S_3.

Accessory Muscles:
GLUTEUS MAXIMUS (Hip extension)
GLUTEUS MEDIUS, POSTERIOR FIBERS (Hip abduction and
  extension)
SARTORIUS (Hip flexion and abduction; knee flexion; knee medial rota-
  tion)

Note: There has long been controversy regarding the rotation action of
the adductors. Some authorities still consider them to be external
rotators with the exception of the vertical fibers of the adductor magnus.

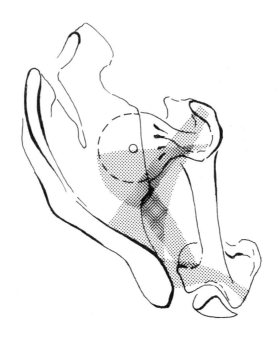

LEFT PELVIS AND FEMUR : SUPERIOR VIEW

Hip Internal Rotation

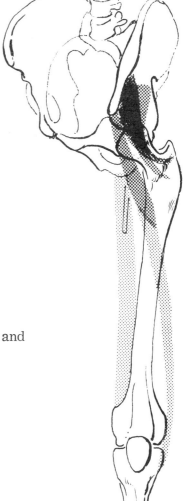

GLUTEUS MEDIUS, ANTERIOR FIBERS (Hip flexion and abduction)

O: Ilium, area between the anterior and the posterior gluteal lines and the crest.
I: Greater trochanter, lateral aspect.
N: Superior gluteal.

GLUTEUS MINIMUS (Hip flexion and abduction)

O: Ilium, area between the anterior and the inferior gluteal lines.
I: Femur, greater trochanter, anterior aspect.
N: Superior gluteal.

TENSOR FASCIA LATAE (Hip flexion and abduction; knee lateral rotation)

O: Iliac crest, anterior part of the outer surface.
I: Iliotibial band, which attaches to the anterior aspect of the lateral tibial condyle.
N: Superior gluteal.

Accessory Muscle:
ADDUCTOR MAGNUS, VERTICAL FIBERS (Hip adduction and extension)

Note: Most authorities now believe that the adductors are weak internal rotators of the hip.

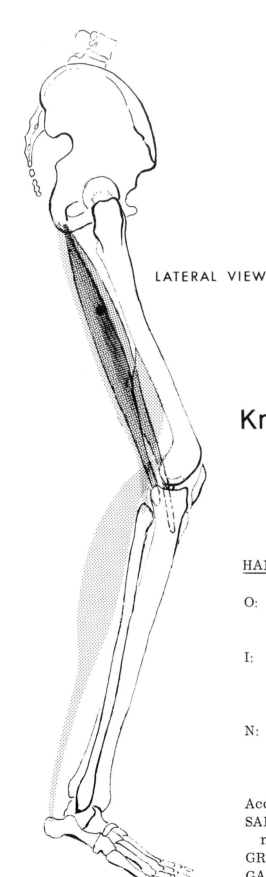

LATERAL VIEW

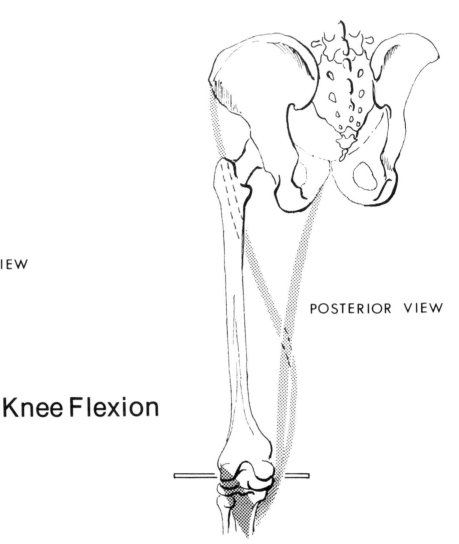

POSTERIOR VIEW

Knee Flexion

HAMSTRINGS (Hip extension; knee rotation)

O: SEMIMEMBRANOSUS, SEMITENDINOSUS, BICEPS
   FEMORIS, LONG HEAD — ischial tuberosity. BICEPS
   FEMORIS, SHORT HEAD — linea aspera, lower part.
I: SEMIMEMBRANOSUS — tibia, posterior surface of the
   medial condyle. SEMITENDINOSUS — tibia, anterior
   surface of the medial condyle. BICEPS FEMORIS — head
   of the fibula.
N: SEMIMEMBRANOSUS, SEMITENDINOSUS, BICEPS
   FEMORIS, LONG HEAD — sciatic, tibial division. BICEPS
   FEMORIS, SHORT HEAD — sciatic, peroneal division。

Accessory Muscles:
SARTORIUS (Hip flexion, abduction and external rotation; knee
   medial rotation)
GRACILIS (Hip adduction; knee medial rotation)
GASTROCNEMIUS (Ankle plantar flexion)
PLANTARIS (Ankle plantar flexion)
POPLITEUS (Knee medial rotation)
O: Femur, lateral epicondyle。
I: Tibia, popliteal line.
N: Tibial.

Knee Rotation

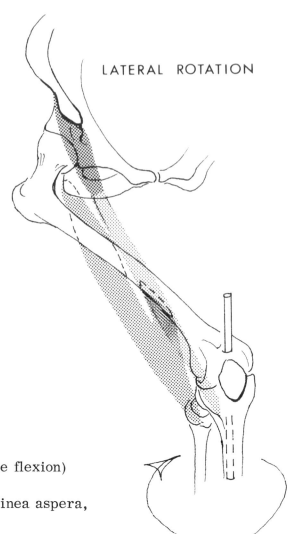

LATERAL ROTATION

Lateral Rotation

BICEPS FEMORIS (Hip extension — long head; knee flexion)

O: Long head — ischial tuberosity; short head — linea aspera,
   lower part.
I: Head of the fibula.
N: Long head — tibial division of the sciatic; short head — peroneal
   division of the sciatic.

Accessory Muscles:
TENSOR FASCIA LATAE (Hip flexion and internal rotation)

Medial Rotation

SEMIMEMBRANOSUS (Hip extension; knee flexion)

O: Ischial tuberosity.
I: Tibia, posterior surface of the medial condyle.
N: Tibial division of the sciatic.

SEMITENDINOSUS (Hip extension; knee flexion)

O: Ischial tuberosity.
I: Tibia, anterior surface of the medial condyle.
N: Tibial division of the sciatic.

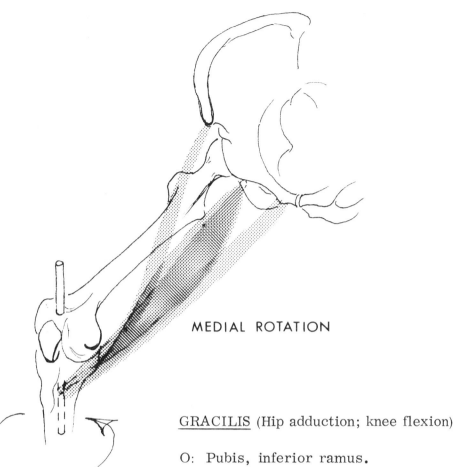

MEDIAL ROTATION

GRACILIS (Hip adduction; knee flexion)

O: Pubis, inferior ramus.
I: Tibia, anterior surface of the medial condyle.
N: Obturator.

POPLITEUS (Knee flexion)

O: Femur, lateral epicondyle.
I: Tibia, popliteal line.
N: Tibial.

SARTORIUS (Hip flexion, abduction and external rotation; knee
   flexion)

O: Anterior superior iliac spine.
I: Tibia, anterior surface of the medial condyle.
N: Femoral.

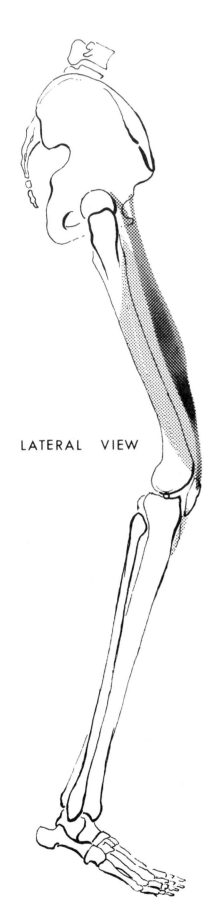

LATERAL VIEW

Knee Extension

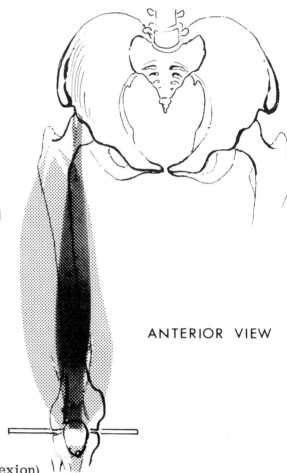

ANTERIOR VIEW

RECTUS FEMORIS (Hip flexion)

O: Straight head — anterior inferior iliac spine; reflected head — superior rim of the acetabulum.
I: Patella and tibial tuberosity via the patellar ligament.
N: Femoral.

VASTUS LATERALIS

O: Femur, intertrochanteric line and linea aspera.
I: Patella and tibial tuberosity via the patellar ligament.
N: Femoral.

VASTUS MEDIALIS

O: Femur, linea aspera.
I: Patella and tibial tuberosity via the patellar ligament.
N: Femoral.

VASTUS INTERMEDIUS

O: Femoral shaft, upper part of the anterior aspect.
I: Patella and tibial tuberosity via the patellar ligament.
N: Femoral.

Ankle Dorsiflexion

TIBIALIS ANTERIOR (Inversion of the foot)

O: Tibia, proximal part, lateral surface.
I: First cuneiform and base of the first metatarsal.
N: Deep peroneal.

EXTENSOR HALLUCIS LONGUS (Extension of the great toe)

O: Fibula, middle portion.
I: Great toe, base of the distal phalanx.
N: Deep peroneal.

EXTENSOR DIGITORUM LONGUS (Extension of the lateral four toes;
  eversion of the foot)

O: Tibia, lateral condyle; fibula, superior part, anterolateral aspect.
I: Lateral four toes, base of the distal phalanx.
N: Deep peroneal.

PERONEUS TERTIUS (Eversion of the foot)

O: Fibula, inferior part.
I: Base of the fifth metatarsal.
N: Deep peroneal.

Ankle Plantar Flexion

GASTROCNEMIUS (Knee flexion)

O: Femur, medial and lateral
  epicondyles, posterior
  aspect.
I: Calcaneus, via tendocalcaneus.
N: Tibial.

SOLEUS

O: Fibula, posterior surface,
  superior part;
  tibia, posterior surface,
  popliteal line.
I: Calcaneus, via tendocalcaneus.
N: Tibial.

PLANTARIS (Knee flexion)

O: Femur, lateral epicondyle.
I: Calcaneus, via tendocalcaneus.
N: Tibial.

Accessory Muscles:
FLEXOR HALLUCIS LONGUS (Great
  toe flexion)
O: Fibula, inferior part,
  posterior aspect.
I: Base of distal phalanx,
  great toe.
N: Tibial.

FLEXOR DIGITORUM LONGUS (Toe
  flexion; inversion of the foot)
O: Tibia, middle part,
  posterior aspect.
I: Lateral four toes, base
  of the distal phalanx.
N: Tibial.

TIBIALIS POSTERIOR (Inversion of
  the foot)
PERONEUS LONGUS (Eversion of the foot)
PERONEUS BREVIS (Eversion of the foot)

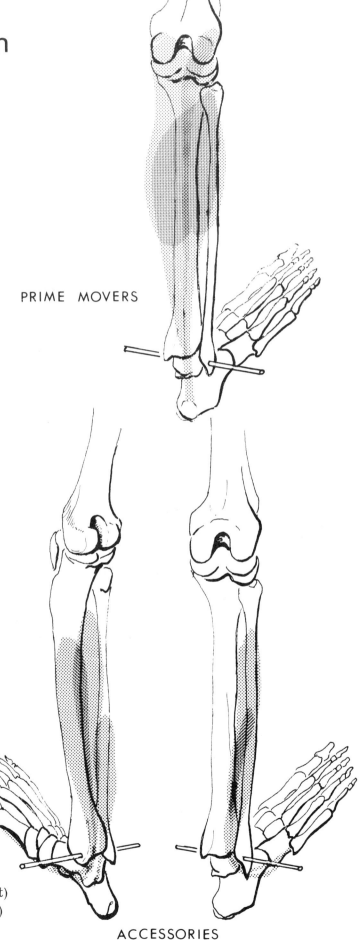

PRIME MOVERS

ACCESSORIES

Foot Inversion

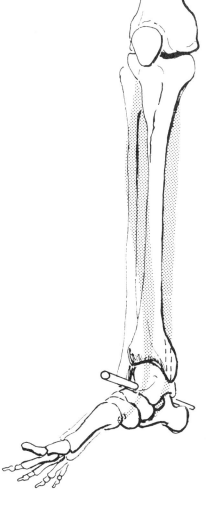

TIBIALIS ANTERIOR (Ankle dorsiflexion)

O: Tibia, superior part, lateral surface.
I: First cuneiform and base of the first metatarsal.
N: Deep peroneal.

TIBIALIS POSTERIOR (Ankle plantar flexion)

O: Tibia and fibula, posterior surface, upper part.
I: All of the tarsal bones except the talus.
N: Tibial.

Accessory Muscle:
FLEXOR DIGITORUM LONGUS (Ankle plantar flexion; toe flexion)
O: Tibia, middle part, posterior surface.
I: Lateral four toes, base of the distal phalanx.
N: Tibial.

Note: Some kinesiologists do not consider the tibialis anterior to be an effective invertor of the foot.

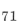

Foot Eversion

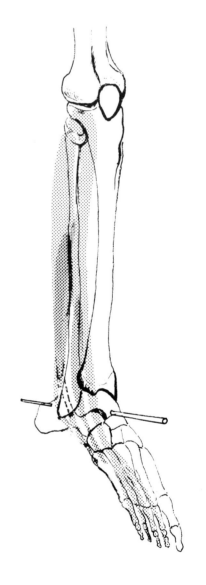

PERONEUS LONGUS (Ankle plantar flexion)

O: Fibula, head and superior part of the lateral aspect.
I: First cuneiform and base of the first metatarsal.
N: Superficial peroneal.

PERONEUS BREVIS (Ankle plantar flexion)

O: Fibula, inferior part of the lateral aspect.
I: Tuberosity of the fifth metatarsal.
N: Superficial peroneal.

PERONEUS TERTIUS (Ankle dorsiflexion)

O: Fibula, inferior part.
I: Base of the fifth metatarsal.
N: Deep peroneal.

EXTENSOR DIGITORUM LONGUS (Ankle dorsiflexion, extension of the
   lateral four toes)

O: Tibia, lateral condyle; fibula, superior part, anterolateral surface.
I: Lateral four toes, base of the distal phalanx.
N: Deep peroneal.

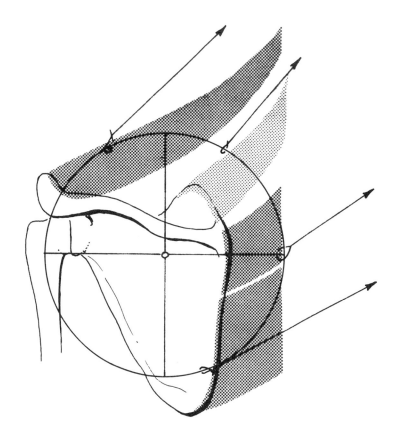

Shoulder Girdle Elevation

TRAPEZIUS, UPPER (Shoulder girdle upward rotation and adduction; neck extension and rotation)

O: Occipital protuberance and ligamentum nuchae.
I: Clavicle, superior surface of the lateral part.
N: Spinal accessory, C_3 and C_4.

LEVATOR SCAPULAE (Shoulder girdle downward rotation)

O: Vertebrae C_1 through C_4.
I: Scapula, medial angle.
N: C_3 and C_4.

RHOMBOIDS, MAJOR AND MINOR (Shoulder girdle adduction and downward rotation)

O: Vertebrae C_7 through T_5.
I: Scapula, vertebral border, from the base of the spine to the inferior angle.
N: Dorsal scapular.

Shoulder Girdle Depression

TRAPEZIUS, LOWER (Shoulder girdle adduction and upward rotation)

O: Vertebrae T_5 through T_{12}.
I: Spine of the scapula, just lateral to the base.
N: Spinal accessory and C_3 and C_4.

LATISSIMUS DORSI (Humeral extension, adduction, and internal rotation)

O: Lower six thoracic and all lumbar vertebrae, sacrum, posterior crest of the ilium, lower three ribs, and inferior angle of the scapula.
I: Humerus, intertubercular groove.
N: Thoracodorsal.

PECTORALIS MAJOR, STERNAL HEAD (Shoulder girdle abduction; shoulder extension, adduction, horizontal adduction, and internal rotation)

O: Sternum and costal cartilages of the upper six ribs.
I: Humerus, intertubercular groove.
N: Medial and lateral pectoral.

PECTORALIS MINOR (Shoulder girdle downward rotation and abduction)

O: Ribs 3, 4, and 5, near the costal cartilages.
I: Coracoid process.
N: Medial pectoral.

Note: Some kinesiologists include the serratus anterior, lower fibers, as a shoulder depressor.

ANTERIOR VIEW

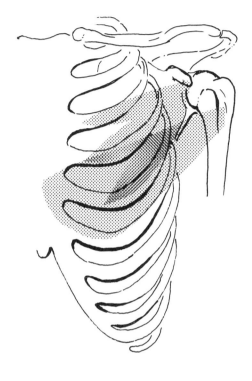

LATERAL VIEW

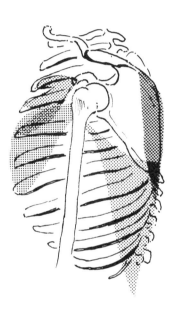

POSTERIOR VIEW

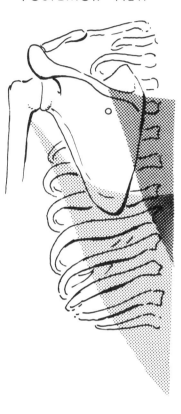

LATERAL VIEW

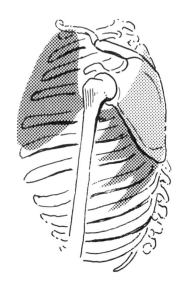

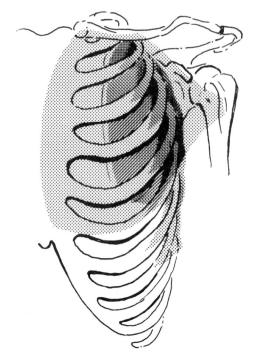

Shoulder Girdle Abduction

SERRATUS ANTERIOR (Upward rotation)

O: Upper eight or nine ribs, lateral aspect.
I: Scapula, anterior surface of the medial border.
N: Long thoracic.

PECTORALIS MAJOR (Shoulder girdle abduction and depression;
   shoulder internal rotation, adduction, flexion — clavicular head;
   and extension — sternal head)

O: Clavicular head — clavicle, medial part.
    Sternal head — sternum and costal cartilages of the upper six ribs.
I: Humerus, intertubercular groove.
N: Medial and lateral pectoral.

PECTORALIS MINOR (Shoulder girdle depression and downward
   rotation)

O: Ribs 3, 4, and 5, near the costal cartilages.
I: Coracoid process.
N: Medial pectoral.

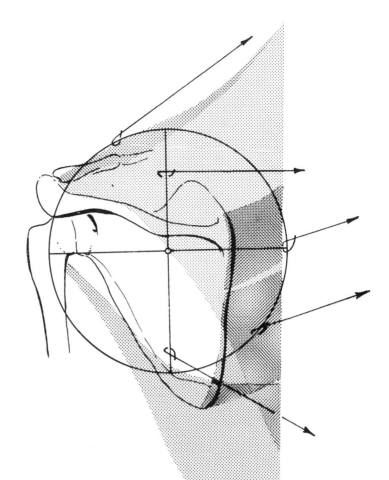

Shoulder Girdle Adduction

TRAPEZIUS (Upper — neck extension and rotation; shoulder girdle
  elevation and upward rotation. Lower — shoulder girdle depression
  and upward rotation)

O: Occipital protuberance, ligamentum nuchae, and vertebrae C_7
  through T_{12}.
I: Clavicle, superior surface of the lateral part; scapula, acromion
  and spine, just lateral to the base.
N: Spinal accessory, C_3 and C_4.

RHOMBOIDS, MAJOR AND MINOR (Shoulder girdle elevation and downward rotation)

O: Vertebrae C_7 through T_5.
I: Scapula, vertebral border from the base of the spine to the inferior
  angle.
N: Dorsal scapular.

Note: The latissimus dorsi may also adduct the scapula if it is attached
to the inferior angle.

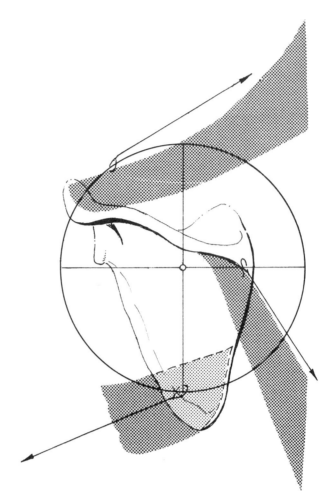

Shoulder Girdle Upward Rotation

SERRATUS ANTERIOR (Shoulder girdle abduction)

O: Lateral aspect of the upper eight or nine ribs.
I: Scapula, anterior surface of the medial border.
N: Long thoracic.

TRAPEZIUS, UPPER (Shoulder girdle elevation and adduction; neck
   extension and rotation)

O: Occipital protuberance and ligamentum nuchae.
I: Clavicle, superior aspect of the lateral part.
N: Spinal accessory, C_3 and C_4.

TRAPEZIUS, LOWER (Shoulder girdle depression and adduction)

O: Vertebrae T_5 through T_{12}.
I: Scapular spine, just lateral to the base.
N: Spinal accessory, C_3 and C_4.

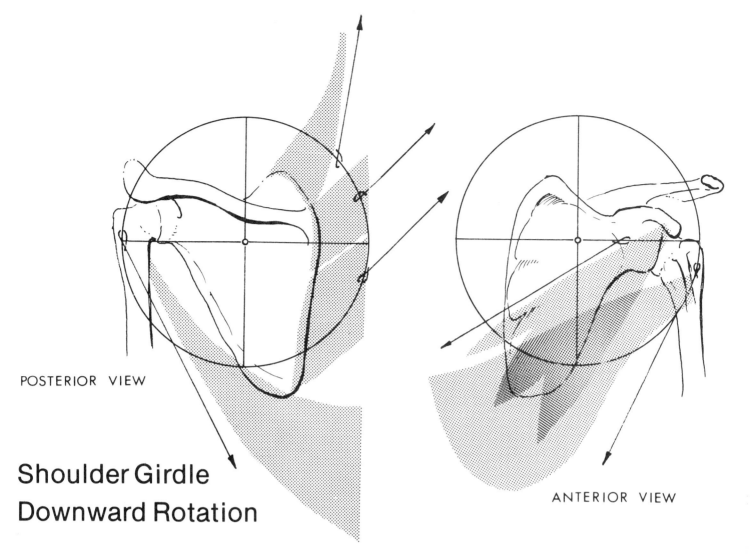

POSTERIOR VIEW

ANTERIOR VIEW

Shoulder Girdle
Downward Rotation

LEVATOR SCAPULAE (Shoulder girdle elevation)

O: Vertebrae C_1 through C_4.
I: Scapula, medial angle.
N: C_3 and C_4.

RHOMBOIDS, MAJOR AND MINOR
   (Shoulder girdle elevation and adduction)

O: Vertebrae C_7 through T_5.
I: Scapula, vertebral border from the base
   of the spine to the inferior angle.
N: Dorsal scapular.

PECTORALIS MINOR (Scapular depression and abduction)

O: Ribs 3, 4, and 5, near the costal cartilages.
I: Coracoid process.
N: Medial pectoral.

Note: The latissimus dorsi,
through its attachments on the
scapula and the humerus, and
the pectoralis major, sternal
head, through its attachment
on the humerus, are considered
by some authors to be downward
rotators of the shoulder girdle.

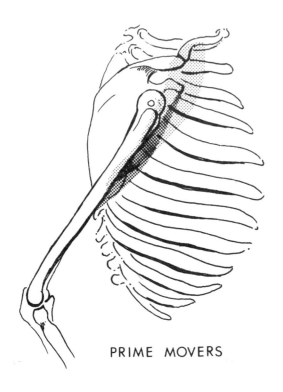

PRIME MOVERS

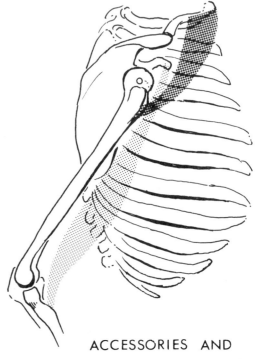

ACCESSORIES AND
PECTORALIS MAJOR : CLAVICULAR HEAD

Shoulder Flexion

ANTERIOR DELTOID (Shoulder abduction, horizontal adduction, and
   internal rotation)

O: Clavicle, lateral part.
I: Humerus, deltoid tuberosity.
N: Axillary.

CORACOBRACHIALIS (Shoulder adduction and horizontal adduction)

O: Coracoid process.
I: Humerus, middle part of the medial aspect.
N: Musculocutaneous.

PECTORALIS MAJOR, CLAVICULAR HEAD (Shoulder girdle abduction;
   shoulder adduction, horizontal adduction, and internal rotation)

O: Clavicle, medial part.
I: Humerus, intertubercular groove.
N: Lateral pectoral.

Accessory Muscles:
BICEPS BRACHII (Elbow flexion; forearm supination; shoulder adduction
   and horizontal adduction — short head)

Shoulder Extension

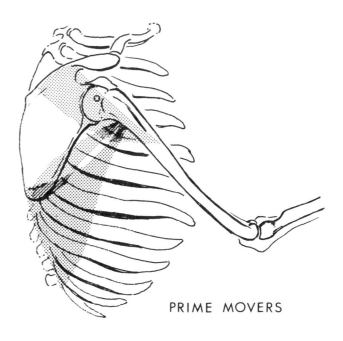

PRIME MOVERS

POSTERIOR DELTOID (Shoulder abduction,
  horizontal abduction, and external rotation)

O: Spine of the scapula.
I: Humerus, deltoid tuberosity.
N: Axillary.

TERES MAJOR (Shoulder adduction and internal rotation)

O: Scapula, dorsal surfaces of the inferior angle.
I: Humerus, intertubercular groove.
N: Lower subscapular.

LATISSIMUS DORSI (Shoulder girdle depression;
  shoulder adduction and internal rotation)

O: Lower six thoracic and all lumbar vertebrae, sacrum, posterior crest of the ilium, lower three ribs,
   and inferior angle of the scapula.
I: Humerus, intertubercular groove.
N: Thoracodorsal.

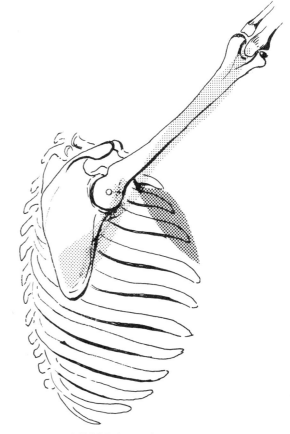

PECTORALIS MAJOR, STERNAL HEAD (Shoulder
  girdle abduction and depression; shoulder adduction,
  horizontal adduction, and internal rotation)

O: Sternum and costal cartilages of the upper six ribs.
I: Humerus, intertubercular groove.
N: Medial and lateral pectoral.

ACCESSORIES AND
PECTORALIS MAJOR : STERNAL HEAD

Accessory Muscles:
INFRASPINATUS, LOWER FIBERS (Shoulder external rotation and
  horizontal abduction)
TERES MINOR (Shoulder external rotation and horizontal abduction)
TRICEPS, LONG HEAD (Shoulder adduction; elbow extension)

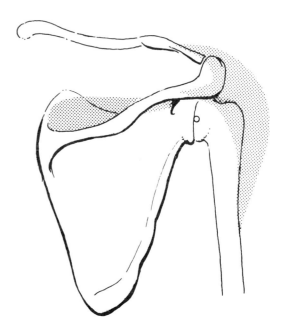

Shoulder Abduction

MIDDLE DELTOID

O: Scapula, acromion process.
I: Humerus, deltoid tuberosity.
N: Axillary.

SUPRASPINATUS

O: Scapula, supraspinous fossa.
I: Humerus, superior facet of the greater tubercle.
N: Suprascapular.

Accessory Muscles:
ANTERIOR DELTOID (Shoulder flexion, horizontal adduction, and internal rotation)
POSTERIOR DELTOID (Shoulder extension, horizontal abduction, and external rotation)

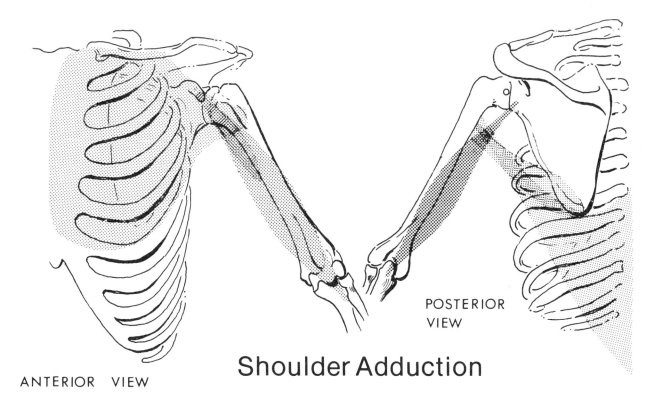

ANTERIOR VIEW

POSTERIOR
VIEW

Shoulder Adduction

PECTORALIS MAJOR (Shoulder girdle abduction and depression; shoulder internal rotation, horizontal adduction, flexion — clavicular head; and extension — sternal head)

O: Clavicular head — clavicle, medial part. Sternal head — sternum and costal cartilages of the upper six ribs.
I: Humerus, intertubercular groove.
N: Medial and lateral pectoral.

TERES MAJOR (Shoulder extension and internal rotation)

O: Scapula, dorsal surface of the inferior angle.
I: Humerus, intertubercular groove.
N: Lower subscapular.

LATISSIMUS DORSI (Shoulder girdle depression; shoulder extension and internal rotation)

O: Lower six thoracic and all lumbar vertebrae, sacrum, posterior crest of the ilium, lower three ribs, and inferior angle of the scapula.
I: Humerus, intertubercular groove.
N: Thoracodorsal.

Accessory Muscles:
TRICEPS, LONG HEAD (Shoulder extension; elbow extension)
CORACOBRACHIALIS (Shoulder flexion and horizontal adduction)
BICEPS BRACHII, SHORT HEAD (Shoulder flexion and horizontal adduction; elbow flexion; forearm supination)

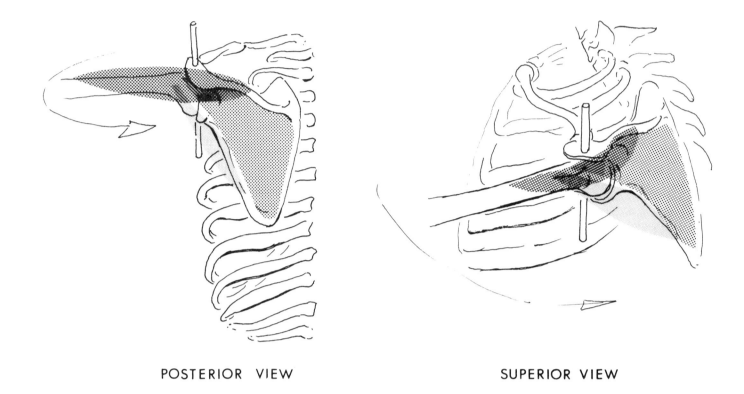

POSTERIOR VIEW   SUPERIOR VIEW

Shoulder Horizontal Abduction

<u>POSTERIOR DELTOID</u> (Shoulder abduction, extension, and external rotation)

O: Spine of the scapula.
I: Humerus, deltoid tuberosity.
N: Axillary.

Accessory Muscles:
INFRASPINATUS (Shoulder external rotation and extension)
TERES MINOR (Shoulder external rotation and extension)

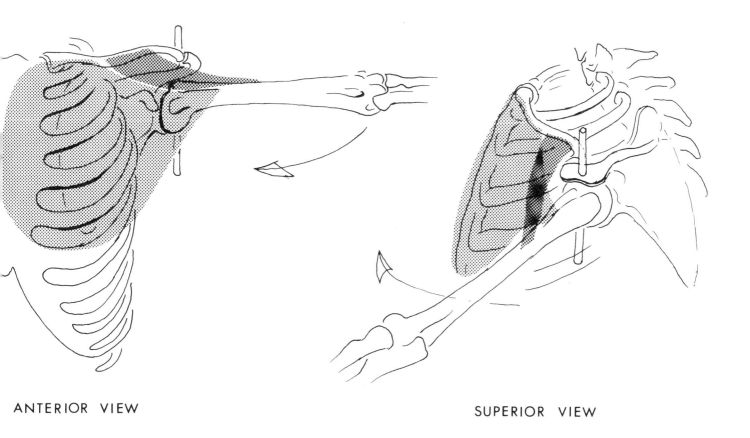

ANTERIOR VIEW   SUPERIOR VIEW

Shoulder Horizontal Adduction

PECTORALIS MAJOR (Shoulder girdle abduction and depression;
  shoulder internal rotation, adduction, flexion — clavicular head;
  and extension — sternal head)

O: Clavicular head — clavicle, medial part; sternal head — sternum
   and costal cartilages of the upper six ribs.
I: Humerus, intertubercular groove.
N: Medial and lateral pectoral.

ANTERIOR DELTOID

O: Clavicle, lateral part.
I: Humerus, deltoid tuberosity.
N: Axillary.

Accessory Muscles:
BICEPS BRACHII, SHORT HEAD (Shoulder flexion and adduction; elbow
  flexion; forearm supination)
CORACOBRACHIALIS (Shoulder flexion and adduction)

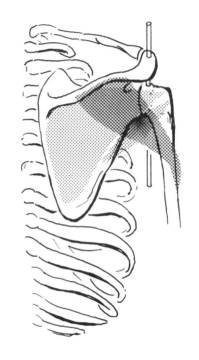

Shoulder External Rotation

INFRASPINATUS (Shoulder extension
   and horizontal abduction)

O: Scapula, infraspinous fossa.
I: Humerus, middle facet of the greater tubercle.
N: Suprascapular.

TERES MINOR (Shoulder extension
   and horizontal abduction)

O: Scapula, upper part of the lateral border.
I: Humerus, inferior facet of the
    greater tubercle.
N: Axillary.

Accessory Muscle:
POSTERIOR DELTOID (Shoulder extension, abduction,
   and horizontal abduction)

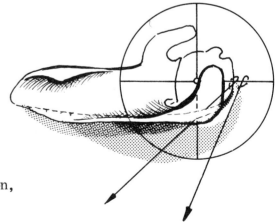

SHOULDER GIRDLE : SUPERIOR VIEW

Shoulder Internal Rotation

SUBSCAPULARIS

O: Subscapular fossa.
I: Humerus, lesser tubercle.
N: Upper and lower subscapular.

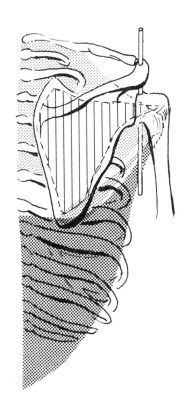

PECTORALIS MAJOR (Shoulder girdle abduction and depression; shoulder adduction,
   horizontal adduction, flexion — clavicular
   head; and extension — sternal head)

O: Clavicle, medial part; sternum and
   costal cartilages of the upper six ribs.
I: Humerus, intertubercular groove.
N: Medial and lateral pectoral.

LATISSIMUS DORSI (Shoulder girdle depression; shoulder adduction and
   extension)

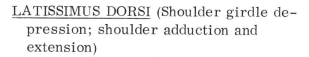

O: Lower six thoracic and all lumbar
   vertebrae, sacrum, posterior crest of
   the ilium, lower three ribs, and inferior
   angle of the scapula.
I: Humerus, intertubercular groove.
N: Thoracodorsal.

TERES MAJOR (Shoulder adduction and
   extension)

O: Scapula, dorsal surface of the inferior
   angle.
I: Humerus, intertubercular groove.
N: Lower subscapular.

Accessory Muscle:
ANTERIOR DELTOID (Shoulder flexion,
   abduction, and horizontal adduction)

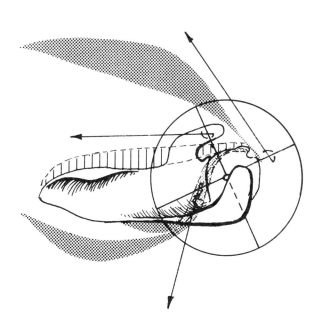

SHOULDER GIRDLE : SUPERIOR VIEW

Elbow Flexion

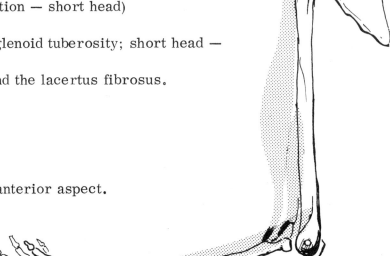

BICEPS BRACHII (Shoulder flexion; forearm supination; shoulder adduction and horizontal adduction — short head)

O: Long head — scapula, supraglenoid tuberosity; short head — scapula, coracoid process.
I: Radius, radial tuberosity, and the lacertus fibrosus.
N: Musculocutaneous.

BRACHIALIS

O: Humerus, lower part of the anterior aspect.
I: Ulnar tuberosity.
N: Musculocutaneous.

BRACHIORADIALIS

O: Humerus, lateral supracondylar ridge.
I: Radius, styloid process.
N: Radial.

Accessory Muscles:
FLEXOR CARPI RADIALIS (Wrist flexion and radial deviation)
FLEXOR DIGITORUM SUPERFICIALIS (Wrist and finger flexion)
PRONATOR TERES (Forearm pronation)
EXTENSOR CARPI RADIALIS LONGUS (Wrist extension and radial deviation)
PALMARIS LONGUS (Wrist flexion)
O: Medial epicondyle, common flexor tendon.
I: Palmar aponeurosis.
N: Median.

Elbow Extension

<u>TRICEPS</u> (Shoulder adduction and extension — long head)

O: Long head — scapula, infraglenoid tuberosity; lateral head —
   humerus, upper part, lateral aspect of the posterior surface;
   medial head — humerus, lower part of the posterior surface.
I: Ulna, olecranon process.
N: Radial.

Accessory Muscle:
ANCONEUS
O: Lateral epicondyle.
I: Olecranon, lateral side.
N: Radial.

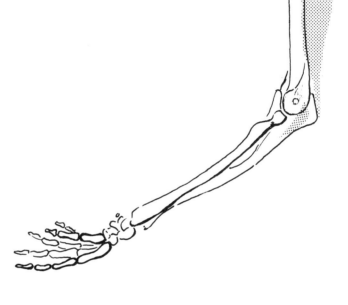

Forearm Pronation

PRONATOR TERES (Elbow flexion)

O: Medial epicondyle, common flexor tendon; ulna, coronoid process.
I: Radius, middle part of the lateral side.
N: Median.

PRONATOR QUADRATUS

O: Ulna, distal part of the anterior surface.
I: Radius, distal part of the anterior surface.
N: Median.

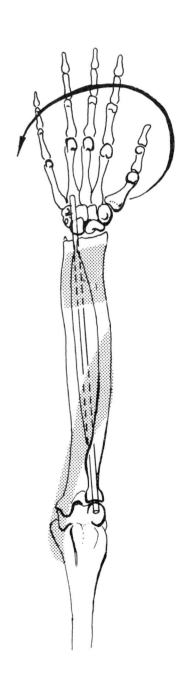

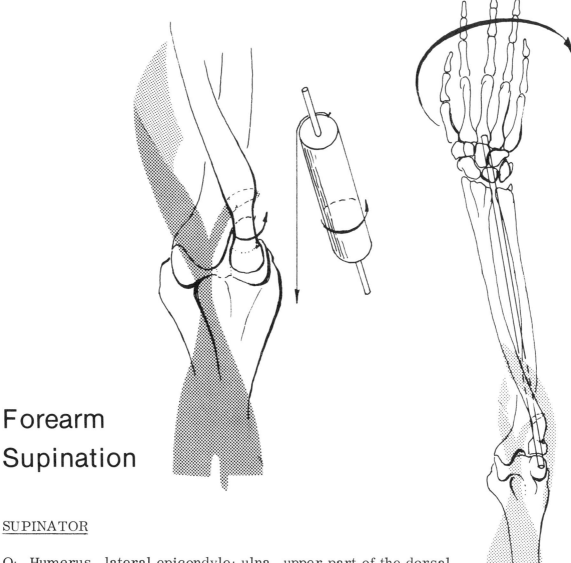

Forearm
Supination

<u>SUPINATOR</u>

O: Humerus, lateral epicondyle; ulna, upper part of the dorsal
   aspect.
I: Radius, upper part of the anterolateral surface.
N: Radial.

<u>BICEPS BRACHII</u> (Shoulder flexion; elbow flexion; shoulder
   adduction and horizontal adduction — short head)

O: Long head — scapula, supraglenoid tuberosity; short head —
   scapula, coracoid process.
I: Radial tuberosity and the lacertus fibrosus.
N: Musculocutaneous.

Note: The left illustration above is an enlarged volar view of the elbow
joint depicting the insertion of the biceps on the radius. The doweling
represents the radius with the arrows illustrating the supinatory effects
of the biceps.

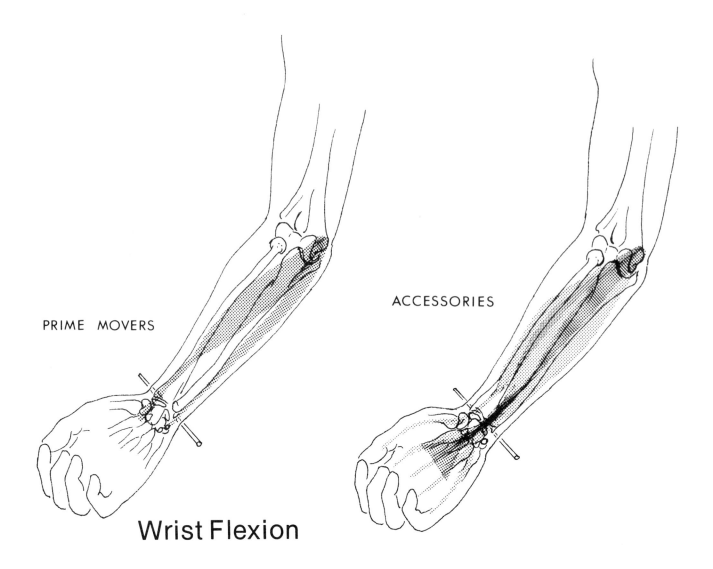

PRIME MOVERS

ACCESSORIES

Wrist Flexion

FLEXOR CARPI RADIALIS (Wrist radial deviation; elbow flexion)

O: Medial epicondyle, common flexor tendon.
I: Base of the second metacarpal.
N: Median.

FLEXOR CARPI ULNARIS (Wrist ulnar deviation)

O: Medial epicondyle, common flexor tendon; ulna, upper part of the dorsal border.
I: Pisiform.
N: Ulnar.

Accessory Muscles:
PALMARIS LONGUS (Elbow flexion)
FLEXOR DIGITORUM SUPERFICIALIS AND PROFUNDUS (Finger flexion)
FLEXOR POLLICIS LONGUS (Thumb flexion)
ABDUCTOR POLLICIS LONGUS (Wrist radial deviation; thumb abduction and extension)

Wrist Extension

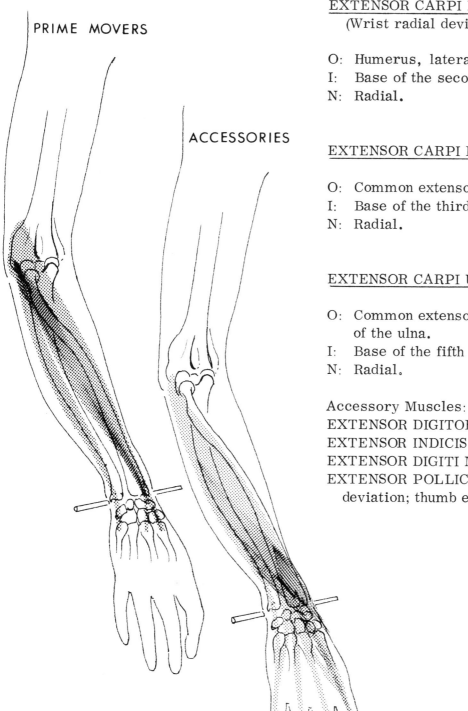

PRIME MOVERS

ACCESSORIES

EXTENSOR CARPI RADIALIS LONGUS
  (Wrist radial deviation; elbow flexion)

O: Humerus, lateral supracondylar ridge.
I: Base of the second metacarpal.
N: Radial.

EXTENSOR CARPI RADIALIS BREVIS

O: Common extensor tendon.
I: Base of the third metacarpal.
N: Radial.

EXTENSOR CARPI ULNARIS (Ulnar deviation)

O: Common extensor tendon and dorsal surface
    of the ulna.
I: Base of the fifth metacarpal.
N: Radial.

Accessory Muscles:
EXTENSOR DIGITORUM (Finger extension)
EXTENSOR INDICIS (Finger extension)
EXTENSOR DIGITI MINIMI (Finger extension)
EXTENSOR POLLICIS LONGUS (Wrist radial
   deviation; thumb extension)

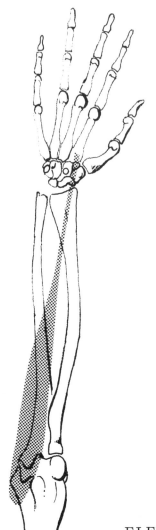

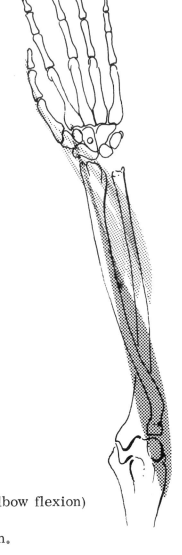

Radial Deviation

FLEXOR CARPI RADIALIS (Wrist flexion; elbow flexion)

O: Medial epicondyle, common flexor tendon.
I: Base of the second metacarpal.
N: Median.

VOLAR VIEW

DORSAL VIEW

EXTENSOR CARPI RADIALIS LONGUS (Wrist extension; elbow
    flexion)

O: Humerus, lateral supracondylar ridge.
I: Base of the second metacarpal.
N: Radial.

Accessory Muscles:
EXTENSOR POLLICIS LONGUS (Wrist extension; thumb extension)
EXTENSOR POLLICIS BREVIS (Thumb extension)
ABDUCTOR POLLICIS LONGUS (Thumb abduction and extension;
    wrist flexion)

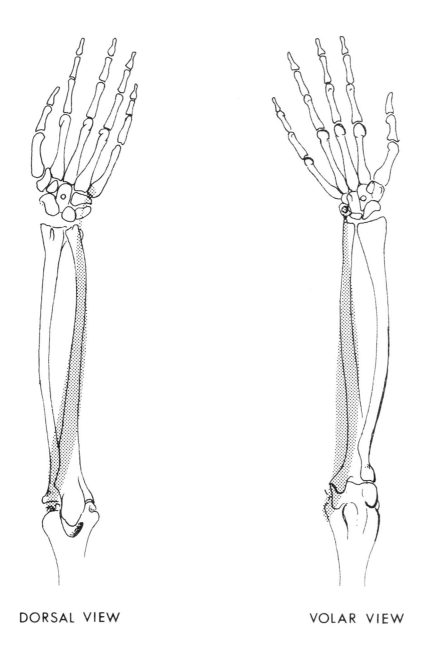

DORSAL VIEW   VOLAR VIEW

Ulnar Deviation

<u>EXTENSOR CARPI ULNARIS</u> (Wrist extension)

O: Common extensor tendon and dorsal surface of the ulna.
I: Base of the fifth metacarpal.
N: Radial.

<u>FLEXOR CARPI ULNARIS</u> (Wrist flexion)

O: Medial epicondyle, common flexor tendon.
I: Pisiform.
N: Ulnar.

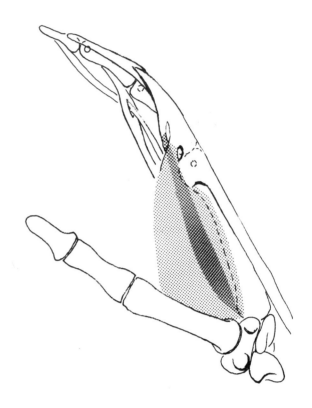

Finger Flexion

Metacarpophalangeal Joint:

INTEROSSEI, DORSAL AND VOLAR (Extension of interphalangeal
   joints; dorsal — finger abduction; volar — finger adduction)

O: Metacarpals.
I: Extensor expansion and base of the proximal phalanx.
N: Ulnar.

LUMBRICALES (Extension interphalangeal joints)

O: Flexor digitorum profundus tendons, radial sides.
I: Extensor expansion, radial side.
N: Median to first and second. Ulnar to third and fourth.

FLEXOR DIGITI MINIMI

O: Hamate and transverse carpal ligament.
I: Base of the proximal phalanx, ulnar side.
N: Ulnar.

Accessory Muscles:
FLEXOR DIGITORUM PROFUNDUS
FLEXOR DIGITORUM SUPERFICIALIS

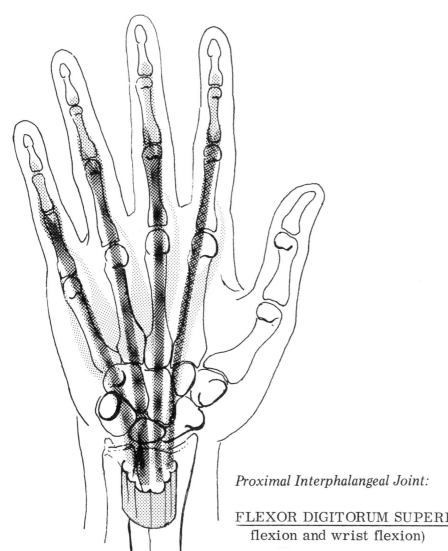

Proximal Interphalangeal Joint:

FLEXOR DIGITORUM SUPERFICIALIS (Metacarpophalangeal
  flexion and wrist flexion)

O: Medial epicondyle, common flexor tendon, ulnar
  coronoid process, oblique line of radius.
I: Medial and lateral sides of the middle phalanx,
  four fingers.
N: Median.

Accessory Muscle:
FLEXOR DIGITORUM PROFUNDUS (Flexion distal phalanx
  fingers and wrist flexion)

Distal Interphalangeal Joint:

FLEXOR DIGITORUM PROFUNDUS (Proximal interphalangeal
  flexion, metacarpophalangeal flexion, and wrist flexion)

O: Upper part of the ulna, anterior surface.
I: Base of distal phalanx, four fingers.
N: Median to index and middle fingers; ulnar to
  ring and little fingers.

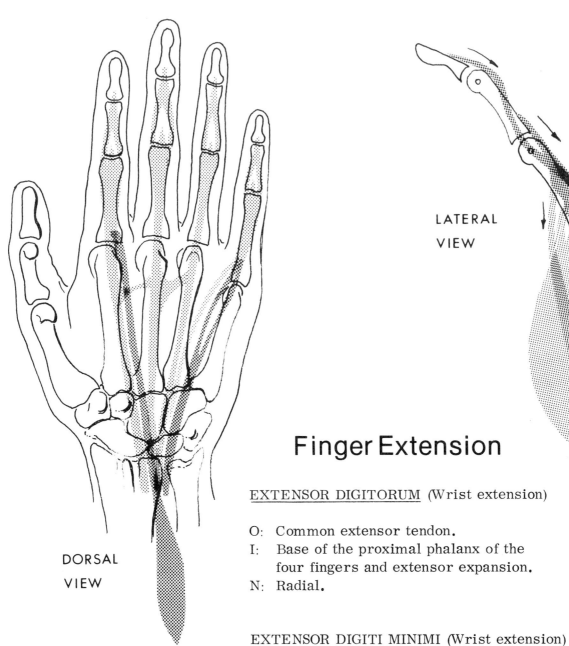

LATERAL
VIEW

DORSAL
VIEW

Finger Extension

EXTENSOR DIGITORUM (Wrist extension)

O: Common extensor tendon.
I: Base of the proximal phalanx of the
four fingers and extensor expansion.
N: Radial.

EXTENSOR DIGITI MINIMI (Wrist extension)

O: Common extensor tendon.
I: Base of the proximal phalanx and exten-
sor expansion, fifth finger.
N: Radial.

EXTENSOR INDICIS (Wrist extension)

O: Distal part of the ulna, dorsal surface.
I: Base of the proximal phalanx and
extensor expansion, index finger.
N: Radial.

LUMBRICALES (Flexion of metacarpophalangeal joints)

O: Flexor digitorum profundus tendons, radial side.
I: Extensor expansion, radial side.
N: Median to first and second; ulnar to third and fourth.

INTEROSSEI, DORSAL AND VOLAR (Flexion of metacarpophalangeal
    joints; dorsal — finger abduction; volar — finger adduction)

O: Metacarpals.
I: Extensor expansion and base of the proximal phalanx, four fingers.
N: Ulnar.

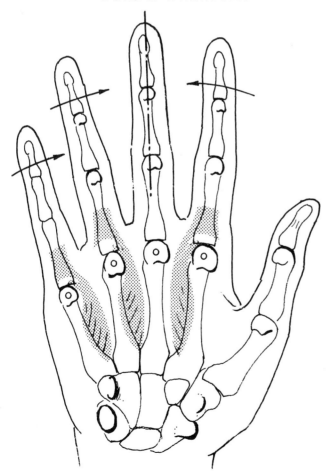

DORSAL INTEROSSEI

VOLAR INTEROSSEI

Finger Abduction

<u>DORSAL INTEROSSEI</u> (Finger flexion —
   metacarpophalangeal joints; and extension
   — interphalangeal joints)

O: Metacarpals, medial and
   lateral surfaces.
I: Extensor expansion and
   base of the proximal phalanges.
N: Ulnar.

<u>ABDUCTOR DIGITI MINIMI</u> (Finger flexion)

O: Pisiform.
I: Base of the proximal phalanx,
   ulnar side, fifth finger.
N: Ulnar.

Finger Adduction

<u>VOLAR INTEROSSEI</u> (Finger flexion —
   metacarpophalangeal joints; and
   extension — interphalangeal joints)

O: Metacarpals, medial or
   lateral surfaces.
I: Extensor expansion and base
   of the proximal phalanges.
N: Ulnar.

Thumb Flexion

Metacarpophalangeal Joint:

FLEXOR POLLICIS BREVIS (Thumb adduction
— deep head)

O: Superficial head — transverse carpal
   ligament and greater multangular;
   deep head — lesser
   multangular and capitate.
I: Thumb, base of the proximal phalanx;
   superficial head — radial side;
   deep head — ulnar side.
N: Superficial head — median;
   deep head — ulnar.

Accessory Muscles:
FLEXOR POLLICIS LONGUS (Thumb
   interphalangeal flexion; wrist flexion)
ABDUCTOR POLLICIS BREVIS (Thumb abduction)

Interphalangeal Joint:

FLEXOR POLLICIS LONGUS (Wrist flexion)

O: Radius, middle part of the
   anterior surface.
I: Thumb, base of the distal phalanx.
N: Median.

Thumb Extension

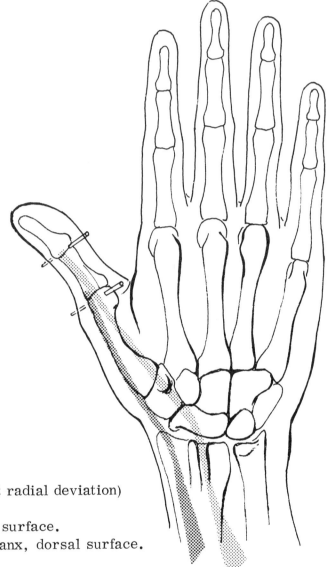

Metacarpophalangeal Joint:

EXTENSOR POLLICIS BREVIS (Wrist radial deviation)

O: Radius, middle part of the dorsal surface.
I: Thumb, base of the proximal phalanx, dorsal surface.
N: Radial.

Accessory Muscles:
ABDUCTOR POLLICIS LONGUS (Wrist flexion
    and radial deviation; thumb abduction)
EXTENSOR POLLICIS LONGUS (Wrist extension
    and radial deviation; extension, thumb
    interphalangeal joint)

Interphalangeal Joint:

EXTENSOR POLLICIS LONGUS (Wrist extension and
    radial deviation)

O: Ulna, middle part of the dorsal surface.
I: Thumb, base of the distal phalanx, dorsal surface.
N: Radial.

Thumb Adduction

ADDUCTOR POLLICIS

O: Oblique head — capitate and bases of the second and third
   metacarpals. Transverse head — body of the third
   metacarpal.
I: Thumb, base of the proximal phalanx, medial side.
N: Ulnar.

Accessory Muscle:
FLEXOR POLLICIS BREVIS, DEEP HEAD (Thumb flexion)

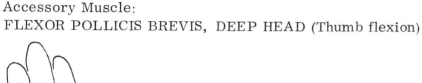

THUMB ADDUCTORS

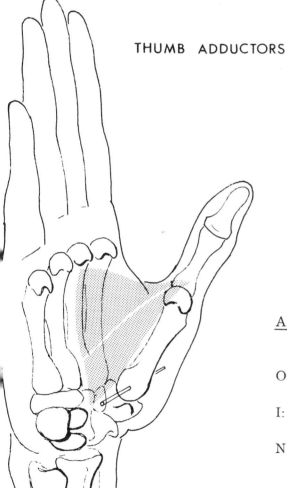

THUMB ABDUCTORS

Thumb Abduction

ABDUCTOR POLLICIS BREVIS (Thumb
   metacarpophalangeal flexion)

O: Greater multangular and transverse
   carpal ligament.
I: Thumb, base of the proximal phalanx,
   lateral side.
N: Median.

ABDUCTOR POLLICIS LONGUS (Wrist radial deviation
   and flexion; thumb extension)

O: Radius and ulna, middle part of the dorsal surface.
I: Thumb, base of the first metacarpal, lateral side.
N: Radial.

103

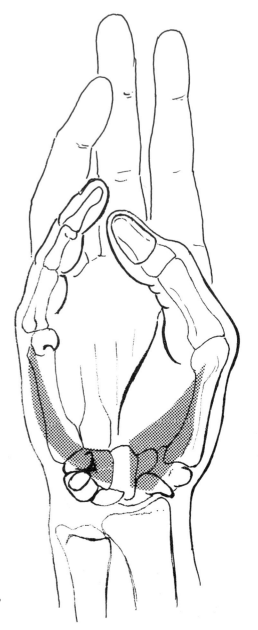

Opposition

OPPONENS POLLICIS

O: Greater multangular and transverse carpal ligament.
I: Thumb, shaft of the metacarpal, radial side.
N: Median.

OPPONENS DIGITI MINIMI

O: Hamate and transverse carpal ligament.
I: Fifth metacarpal, ulnar side of the shaft.
N: Ulnar.

Note: The ability to functionally oppose requires that additional muscles act on the thumb and little finger. The thumb must circumduct, a combination of abduction, rotation, and flexion, at the carpometacarpal joint in order to effectively oppose any of the fingers. Likewise, the little finger must rotate and flex at its carpometacarpal joint.

Problems

These problems are presented to direct your study to the various principles of muscle function and movement. Assignments may be made periodically as the subject matter is pertinent to your study in class. Because this manual begins with the lower extremity and ends with the upper extremity, many of the first problems are related to lower extremity activity. Problems 13 through 25 deal exclusively with the upper extremity.

1. Movement of the human body, like that of a machine, is subject to the law of mechanics. Motion occurs when the force of a contracting muscle is applied to the skeleton, which is actually a system of levers. When several muscles contract, their individual forces are combined into one single force. The motion which occurs depends on the direction of the combined force.

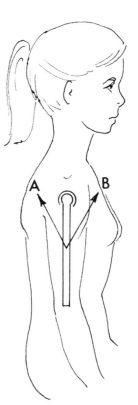

   A and B represent the action lines of two muscles.
   If muscle A contracts, the resulting motion

will be _____ of the
            (flexion/extension)
shoulder joint.
   If muscle B contracts, the resulting motion

of the shoulder joint will be _____.
                              (flexion/extension)
   If the two muscles contract simultaneously their forces will be combined and will result in a different motion. Construct a parallelogram with an arrow designating the direction of the combined force. This combined force will result in a

shoulder motion of _____.
   In mechanics this process is called composition of forces. It is also an example of the synergistic action of muscles.

2. Another process from mechanics which can be related to movement is that of the resolution of forces — resolving a single force into its component parts. This is important in determining the

effectiveness of a muscle's force in causing motion. In most instances a muscle's force has two components — a rotatory force which will cause movement and a nonrotatory force.

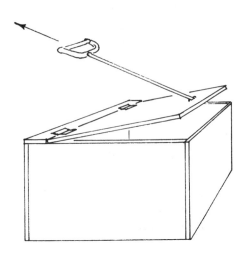

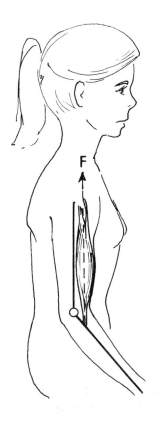

a. When a force is applied to the handle of the box on the left, the lid will open because the hinges provide an axis where rotation can occur. Owing to the angle of the handle only part of the force will be effective in raising, or rotating, the lid. Construct a parallelogram and resolve the force into its two components. Label the rotatory force A and the nonrotatory component B. In this example the rotatory force

is _____ than the
    (greater/less)
nonrotatory force.
How would you position the handle so that the lid could be raised with

the least amount of force? _____

_____

b. Contraction of a muscle for the purpose of causing motion (rotation of the bone around an axis which is in the joint) also results in rotatory and nonrotatory force components. F represents the action line of an elbow flexor muscle. Construct a parallelogram and label the rotatory and nonrotatory components of the force as in the above problem.

At what elbow position would the greatest amount of the force be

applied to rotation? _____

_____

3. Leverage is one of the factors which determines the amount of force required of a contracting muscle. According to the law of levers, force times force arm equals resistance times resistance arm. The amount of force required will be increased if the amount of weight (resistance) is increased or if the length of the resistance arm is increased. Also, the amount of force required may be increased or decreased by changing the length of the force arm. The beater of the loom is an example of a third-class lever which demonstrates changes in force requirements.

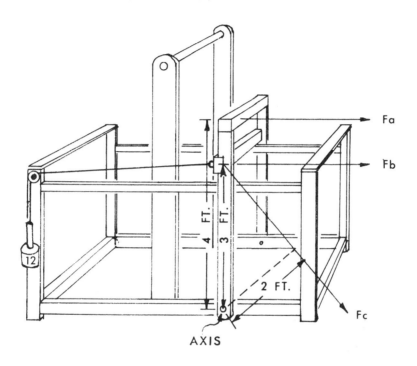

If a resistance of 12 pounds is attached to the beater at a point 3 feet from the axis, the resistance arm (perpendicular distance between the line of action of the resistance and the axis) is 3 feet. If the force Fb is applied to the beater at the same point as the resistance, the force arm is also 3 feet. If we have determined that the amount of force required at Fb is 12 pounds, how much force would be required at Fa and Fc? Note that the force Fc is applied to the beater at an angle less than 90 degrees and that the force arm (perpendicular distance between the line of action of the force and the axis) is 2 feet.

_____ = force required at Fa

_____ = force required at Fc

Forces Fb and Fc are both applied to the beater at a point 3 feet from the axis. Explain why the force required at Fc is greater

than the force required at Fb. _____

_____

If the point of attachment of the resistance were moved up to the top of the beater (at 4 feet) the amount of force required at

Fa would be _____ than in the previous example.
                  (greater/less)

(Note: If we wanted to calculate the exact force requirements, other factors, such as friction and the effects of gravity, should be included in the calculations. The purpose of this problem is to help you understand the concepts of leverage.)

4. With the arm in position A on the figure below, the maximum weight an individual can hold with the elbow flexors is 10 pounds. He

should be able to hold approximately _____ pounds with the arm in position B.

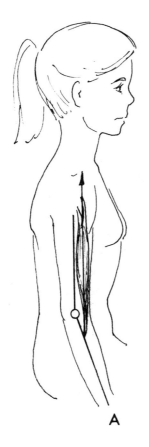 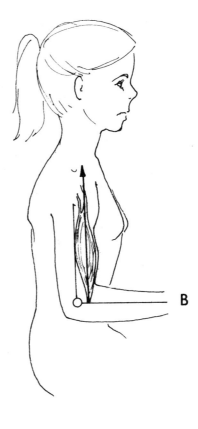

B

A

5. You have found that the maximum weight an individual can lift with the elbow flexors is 15 pounds. If the weights are held in the hand the resistance arm is equivalent to the length of the forearm, which you have measured and found to be 10 inches. How much weight should this individual be able to lift if you increased the resistance arm length to 15 inches by attaching the weights to a 5-inch stick which he holds in the hand while flexing the elbow?

_____ pounds.

If the same individual had an amputation with the end of the stump 5 inches from the elbow joint, he should be able to lift

_____ pounds if the weights are attached to the end of the stump with a strap.

6. A contracting muscle is equally capable of causing movement of either bone to which it is attached. If it is to effectively produce motion of just one of the bones either its proximal or its distal attachment must be anchored or fixated.

a. When the iliopsoas flexes the femur the proximal attachment of the muscle on the pelvis must be fixated by the

_____ muscles.

b. When the desired motion is hip extension, the proximal attachment of the extensor muscles is fixated by the

_____.

c. When you are in a standing position the weight of the body does not allow the legs to move. If, in this position, the right external rotators of the hip contract, the resulting motion will

be rotation of the pelvis to the _____.

d. Place your subject in a supine position on the table with both legs stabilized to prevent movement. What motion will occur

when the hip flexor muscles contract? _____

_____

7. A muscle is capable of applying its greatest force when it is at its maximum length or slightly stretched. Also, a muscle's ability to shorten during contraction is limited to approximately 50 percent of its total length. These characteristics must be considered in the analysis of muscle function and have special implications for muscles which cross, and can act on, two joints.

    a. When a bicycler is pedaling up a hill he leans forward at the hip

       joint to place the _____muscle on stretch.

    b. The rectus femoris is capable of applying its greatest force to

       knee extension when the hip joint is in the_____
       position.

    c. The hamstrings will be most effective in producing hip

       extension when the knee is in the _____ position.

    d. While standing on your left leg, flex your right knee with the hip flexed. Now flex your right knee with the hip in the extended

       position. Movement is easier when the hip is_____

       because _____.
       An additional consideration in the analysis above is the fact that when one group of muscles contracts, its opposing, antagonistic, group of muscles is being stretched and may eventually limit motion. When knee flexion is attempted with the hip in maximum

       extension the_____ muscle is being stretched and may
       limit the motion.

8. The majority of our muscles are capable of producing more than one action at a joint. When only one of a muscle's possible actions is desired, synergistic action is usually required to neutralize the undesired motions. The gluteus medius is capable of producing five

       different motions at the hip joint which are _____ .
       How do its anterior and posterior fibers act synergistically when

       hip abduction is the desired motion? _____

9. Muscles are capable of contracting concentrically (a shortening contraction) or eccentrically (a lengthening contraction). The eccentric contraction of muscles is often necessary to provide controlled motion and is common when gravity is acting as the prime mover.

  a. When you bend forward to pick up an object from the floor, the motion is occurring primarily at the hip joint and gravity is acting as the prime mover. The motion is controlled by the

     _____ muscles which are contracting

     _____.

  b. An individual with weak hip and knee extensor muscles will have difficulty lowering himself into a chair without using his arms.

     Explain. _____

     _____

  c. A third form of muscular contraction is referred to as isometric contraction. A muscle acting in this manner does so to maintain a part in a stable position. When you stand on the left leg with the right foot lifted from the floor, palpation of the left gluteus medius muscle indicates that it is contracting. Why?_____

     _____

  d. Instruct your subject to step up on a stool with the right leg leading and to step down with the left leg leading and the right leg remaining on the stool. Analyze this activity for the right leg and complete the following:

MOTION	JOINT	MUSCLE GROUPS ACTING	TYPE OF CONTRACTION
Positioning the right foot on the stool	Hip		
	Knee		
	Ankle		
Elevation	Hip		
	Knee		
	Ankle		
Descent	Hip		
	Knee		
	Ankle		

10. Ask your subject to stand erect, maintaining the knees in the extended position. Have him sway slightly forward and backward.

The motion is occurring at the _____ joint. The muscles

which perform the forward motion are _____

_____ and those

performing the backward motion are _____

_____. Stability in
standing requires that the center of gravity be maintained over the
base of support. The muscles you have listed above play an important role in standing balance.

11. If the tibialis anterior and the extensor hallucis longus are paralyzed, dorsiflexion of the ankle may be possible but will be accom-

panied by _____.
                                   (motion)
Analysis of this problem points out the importance of synergistic
action of muscles.

12. The ability of the muscles which plantar flex the ankle to function
effectively will be decreased if the knee is flexed because

_____

_____.

112

13. The rotatory movements of the scapula may be compared to the turning of a wheel as demonstrated on the drawing below.

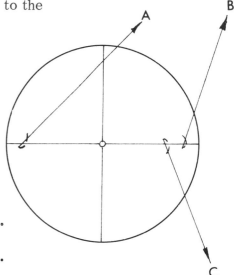

If you pull on rope A the wheel will turn to the _____.

If you pull on rope B the wheel will turn to the _____.

Pulling rope C turns the wheel to the _____.

The muscles which attach to the scapula apply rotatory forces much as the ropes on the wheel.

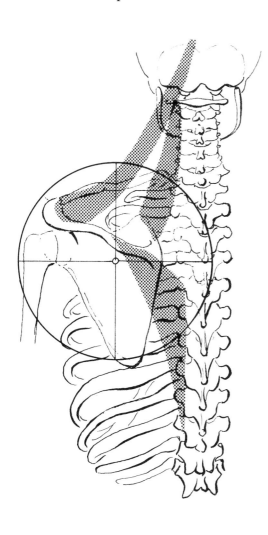

If the levator scapulae contracts,

the scapula will_____ rotate. Contraction of the upper

trapezius will cause_____ rotation. If both the upper and lower trapezius contract, the motion will be

_____ rotation. Combined actions of these muscles will also cause translatory motions of the scapula. If the upper trapezius and levator scapulae contract,

the scapula will_____. Contraction of the lower trapezius and levator scapulae will result in

_____. The latter two motions require the synergistic action of the contracting muscles. Explain.

_____

_____

14. Without the mobility of the shoulder girdle maximal arm motions in the sagittal and coronal planes would be impossible. Because of the mobility, fixation of the shoulder girdle is required if the arm muscles which attach to it are to efficiently apply their force to movement of the humerus.

a. Line A on the diagram below represents the line of force of the infraspinatus and teres minor.

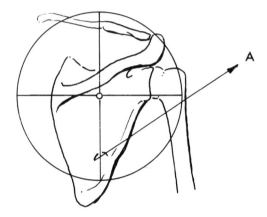

If the fixators are not functioning, contraction of the two

muscles will cause an _____ motion of the shoulder girdle.

On the diagram draw in the force lines of those muscles which can oppose this motion and thus fixate the shoulder girdle.

These shoulder girdle muscles are _____

_____.

b. Line A on the diagram below represents the line of force of the deltoid muscle.

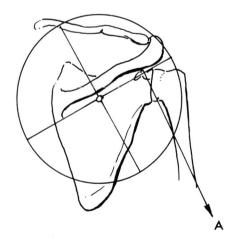

If the fixators are not functioning, contraction of the deltoid

will cause a _____ motion of the shoulder girdle.

On the diagram draw in the force lines of those muscles which can oppose the above motion and thus provide fixation of the shoulder girdle. Label the force lines C, D, and E and name the muscles below.

C _____

D _____

E _____

_____ of the shoulder girdle is
          (motion)
necessary for complete abduction of the arm. This shoulder

girdle motion is provided by _____
muscles.

c. The muscles which fixate the scapula so that the teres major

can apply its force to motion of the humerus are _____

_____.

15. As you perform your activities of daily living, muscles are con-
tinuously lifting your body parts against the effects of gravity.
A muscle possessing sufficient strength to move a body part
against the effects of gravity may be called an antigravity muscle
while one which cannot might be called a nongravity muscle.

a. From a relaxed sitting position, with your hands in your lap,
raise one arm overhead, as you would to ask a question in
class. The muscles acting on the shoulder and elbow primarily responsible for performing this action are

_____.

The motion is being resisted by_____.
As you lower the arm from this overhead position to the mid-

line of the body the motion is performed by _____ .

If you had nongravity muscles and your arm were placed by someone else in the overhead position and then released, what

would happen? _____

Why? _____

If you continue the motion of the arm from the midline of the

body to complete hyperextension the _____

_____muscles contract and the motion is resisted

by _____.

b. Would you expect a person with nongravity muscle strength in the infraspinatus and teres minor to comb the hair on the back

of his head? Explain. _____

_____

16. If all portions of the deltoid muscle function to abduct the shoulder, what synergistic action is necessary?

17. In everyday use of the upper extremities, we commonly reach out and pull back, or return the arm to the proximity of the body. Thus, we commonly use the motions of shoulder flexion with elbow extension and shoulder extension with elbow flexion. Two of the muscles which are active during these motions, and which

cross and can act on both joints, are_____

and _____. How does the motion which is occurring at the shoulder increase the ability of these muscles to apply their force to the elbow motion?

18. What muscles at the shoulder and elbow act when you use a hand-saw to saw through a board?

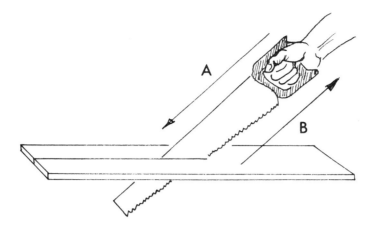

a. On the down stroke (A)? _____

b. On the return stroke (B)? _____

c. In each instance what type of muscular contraction is occurring?

_____

d. What type of muscular contraction is taking place in the finger

flexors as they grip the saw handle? _____

_____

19. Will elbow flexion be possible for a person who has had a severance

of the musculocutaneous nerve? Explain. _____

_____

20. a. Have someone firmly grasp a piece of doweling which measures from 1 inch to 2 inches in diameter with the wrist in a normal dorsiflexed position. Try to pull the piece of doweling from his grasp. Next have your subject firmly grasp the doweling with his wrist in maximum palmar flexion. (Make certain that he maintains his wrist in palmar flexion as he holds the dowel.) Try removing the piece of doweling.

Results of your experiment: _____

_____

_____

_____

b. Using a dynamometer, test and record your subject's grasp strength. Compare this figure with his strength when the wrist is passively held in about 30 degrees of flexion.

Normal grasp strength _____

Grasp strength with wrist flexed _____

c. Wrist position is extremely important for efficient use of the hand. If a person has a hand disabled in a position of palmar

flexion, his grasp strength will be _____
                                      (increased/decreased)

because _____ .

21. With the forearm pronated and resting on the table, forcefully extend the thumb. Palpate the tendon of the extensor carpi ulnaris.

Why is it contracting? _____

_____

22. How do the flexor carpi ulnaris and the flexor carpi radialis

act synergistically during flexion of the wrist? _____

_____

118

23. When you abduct the fifth finger, palpation of the flexor carpi

   ulnaris indicates that it is contracting. Why? _____

   _____

24. List the muscles required to hold a pencil for writing.

   Thumb Muscles: _____

   _____

   Index and Middle Finger Muscles: _____

   _____

25. What muscles are necessary for lateral opposition (placing the pad
   of the thumb against the lateral side of the index finger)?

   Thumb Muscles: _____

   _____

   Index Finger Muscles: _____

   _____

REFERENCES AND INDEX

/

References

Brunnstrom S: Clinical Kinesiology, 3rd ed. Philadelphia, F. A. Davis Company, 1972.

Daniels MA, Worthingham C: Muscle Testing, Techniques of Manual Examination, 3rd ed. Philadelphia, W. B. Saunders Company, 1972.

Grant JCB: An Atlas of Anatomy, 5th ed. Philadelphia, The Wilkins Company, 1962.

Gray H: Anatomy of the Human Body, 27th ed., edited by CM Goss. Philadelphia, Lea and Febiger, 1959.

Hamilton WJ, Simon G: Surface and Radiological Anatomy, 4th ed. Cambridge, W. Heffer and Sons Limited, 1958.

Hollinshead WH: Functional Anatomy of the Limbs and Back, 3rd ed. Philadelphia, W. B. Saunders Company, 1969.

Lampe EW: Surgical Anatomy of the Hand in Clinical Symposia, Vol. 9, No. 1. Summit, N.J., CIBA Products Inc., 1957.

Muscle Function Tests and Measurements, Laboratory Manual. Course in Physical Therapy, University of Minnesota.

Wells KF: Kinesiology: The Scientific Basis of Human Motion, 5th ed. Philadelphia, W. B. Saunders Company, 1971.

Williams M, Lissner HR: Biomechanics of Human Motion. Philadelphia, W. B. Saunders Company, 1962.

Index

124